VETERINARY DENTISTRY

VETERINARY DENTISTRY

Dr. Erich Eisenmenger
Dr. Karl Zetner
Surgical Clinic and Eye Clinic of Veterinary Medicine
University of Vienna, Austria

With the Assistance of
Professor Franz Schütz and
Ben H. Colmery, III, D.V.M.
Executive Director
Society of Veterinary Dentistry

200th Anniversary
1785 – 1985

LEA & FEBIGER

Philadelphia 1985

Lea & Febiger
600 Washington Square
Philadelphia, PA 19106-4198
U.S.A.
(215) 922-1330

Library of Congress Cataloging in Publication Data

Eisenmenger, Erich.
Veterinary dentistry.

Translation of: Tierärztliche Zahnheilkunde.
Includes index.
1. Veterinary dentistry. I. Zetner, Karl.
II. Colmery, Ben H. III. Title.
SF867.E3713 1984 636.089'76 84-7908
ISBN 0-8121-0924-4

PRINTED IN THE UNITED STATES OF AMERICA

Print No. 4 3 2 1

Preface

For many decades, the veterinary treatment of animal's teeth was limited to cleaning, correction of simple functional abnormalities, and extraction. Only a few specialists attempted to pursue the particular problems of veterinary dentistry or to appropriate human dental methods for use on veterinary patients, usually done under the supervision of a dentist or a dental technician. Accordingly, informative publications on the subject of veterinary dentistry were few and far between and difficult for the general practitioner to obtain. Even in the university environment, there was only enough information for sporadic inclusion of veterinary dentistry in clinical, research, and teaching settings.

This obvious omission of a technically interesting and medically important subject motivated us at the Vienna Veterinary Surgery Clinic to add a veterinary dentistry unit for large and small animals to our facility in 1970. Under the direction of Dr. J. Bodingbauer, our clinic has established a tradition of veterinary dentistry, and with the technical expertise of this book's co-author, who is the head of the dentistry unit, the practice of veterinary dentistry has been transformed into a scientific discipline.

In this book, which is the first comprehensive text of veterinary dentistry, we have brought together the knowledge gained through years of experience and the significant points of other authors' writings about tooth development, anatomy, histology, and nomenclature.

We would like to thank our illustrious teacher and former director of our clinic, Dr. Otto Uberreiter, who inspired this book's primary author, a dentist's son, to pursue this field of study, and who passed onto his students a solid training in surgery. We must thank Verlag Paul Parey for being so wonderful to work with, as well as our colleagues at the clinic, who share much of the credit for this book's success.

Vienna

Erich Eisenmenger
Karl Zetner

Contents

1

The Dental Patient

Before starting treatment, each patient should receive a general examination. During prolonged periods of treatment, a general examination should be repeated at intervals of several weeks and always before the patient undergoes anesthesia or surgical procedures.

Special attention should be paid to the patient's nutritional status, regional lymph nodes, heart, circulation, kidney function, and respiration. If required, hematologic studies should be done and blood urea nitrogen and urinary albumin and sediment levels should be determined. The patient's medical history should include the type and duration of possible symptoms, preliminary treatment, and above all, the nature of the food ingested and the characteristics of digestion. Premedication of the patient may be necessary before starting dental treatment.

Teeth and gums should be examined briefly before any veterinary therapy, such as vaccination, is undertaken. The owners of animals are always interested in information on mouth odor, looseness of teeth, and similar findings, and they respond gratefully to reasonable suggestions for treatment.

If the patient is cooperative and if trained auxiliary personnel are at hand, many animals can undergo simple, short-term treatment without sedation or anesthesia. Such simple procedures include the examination of the mouth cavity, the removal of plaque and extremely loose teeth, the polishing of fillings, the abrasion of sharp edges and other superficial irregularities in horses and dogs, and the adjustment of orthodontic appliances.

Restless animals such as cats have to be tranquilized or anesthetized. In such patients, atropine effects the desired inhibition of salivary secretion.

Techniques of anesthesia induction and anesthetic agents are covered adequately in other texts and are not discussed here.

2

Tooth and Jaw

EMBRYOLOGY AND GROWTH

The ectodermal element (dental lamina) originates in the oral epithelium and extends into the mesenchyme, forming the deciduous tooth buds. Also present is an embryonic ectodermal element that soon becomes rudimentary in the os incisivum of cattle; a cornified masticatory plate later develops in place of the upper incisors.

The colloidal enamel pulp of the tooth buds is turned toward the jaw by the mesenchymal papilla; the dental pulp is formed in this cavity. Stratiform odontoblasts begin to secrete dentin at the point of the papilla from which the crown of the tooth develops. The ameloblasts, which are close to the cup-shaped crown, form hexagonal calcifying enamel prisms held together by a cementing substance. The surrounding mesenchyme forms the dental sac and, a short distance away, the alveolar bone. Once the crown of the tooth has been formed, a tubular lamellar enamel grows from the ring-shaped papillary opening into the mesenchyme of the dental sac, and the root begins to develop. Along the tubular lamellar enamel, ameloblasts start to grow from the crown toward the apex of the root and strengthen the roots by the formation of dentin. Thus, the lamellar enamel determines the shape and size of the future tooth. Aberrant teeth, therefore, are primarily misplaced enamel germs. No enamel is producccd by the root's epithelial sheath, which is destroyed by the odontoblasts of the dental sac immediately after birth, when the osteoid cementum firmly combines with the dentin in the root. The outer wall of the dental sac develops into the periodontal ligament, and the inner wall develops into the root cementum.

In complex cuspal enamel teeth, the formation of dentin starts at several papilla points; multirooted teeth are cleft by the epithelial sheath of the enamel pulp, and several isolated cylindric cavities (roots) develop (Fig. 2–1).

The long crowns of herbivores' teeth consist of enamel folds that run parallel to the tooth's center line and form a cylindric cavity open at the end that is in the jaw (Figs. 2–2 and 2–3). The end of the cylinder that is in the oral cavity is closed in certain molars in horses and cattle. The outer cavities of the crown as well as the enamel grooves are filled by cementum. Although the softer ce-

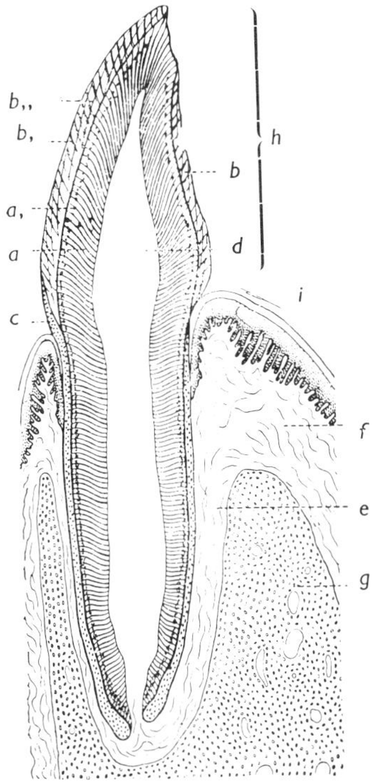

Fig. 2–1. Longitudinal section through an incisor of a cow; natural position in jaw, with the lingual surface to the right. *a* = dentin with dentin canals; *a,* = interglobular dentin; *b* and *b,* and *b,,* = enamel with Schreger's lines; *c* = cementum; *d* = pulp cavity at upper part of root; *e* = alveolar dental cuticle; *f* = gingiva; *g* = mandible; *h* = tooth crown; *i* = cornified epithelial ridge. (From Krölling O, Grau H. Lehrbuch der Histologie und vergleichenden mikroskopischen Anatomie der Haustiere. Berlin: Paul Parey, 1960.)

mentum and dentin are abraded more quickly, the map-like enamel fissures in the occlusal surfaces of molars are developed. The dental pulp is found in one or more root canals which are constantly reduced in size by the formation of secondary dentin of the odontoblasts. The mandibular molars are slender and have two roots; the upper posterior teeth have a cross-cut shape and three roots.

A short time after root formation, tooth eruption and elongation are completed in humans, carnivores, and pigs. The originally wide pulp cavity is progressively contracted by the formation of secondary dentin. Only a fine root canal at the apex of the root is left for the nerves and blood vessels. The contraction of the pulp cavity starts at the crown and is completed in dogs by about 24 months. The reduction in length is insignificant and is partly compensated by involution of the alveolar wall in older animals.

The greater abrasion of herbivores' teeth, which occurs at a rate of about 2.2 mm per year, is compensated by active elongation up to the sixth to eighth year of life; secondary dentin develops, and the pulp recedes. Later, toward the end of the active elongation, 1 to 3 short, curved roots develop without enamel. These roots contain the thin root canal. Because of the further deposition of secondary dentin and cementum over the course of 18 to 20 years, the root becomes necrotic, and the tooth dies.

The reduction in length caused by abrasion is compensated until about the

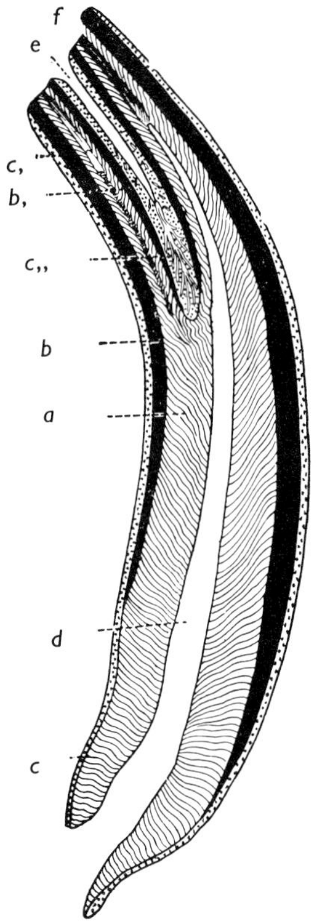

Fig. 2–2. Longitudinal section through an incisor in horse, natural size. *a* = dentin with canals; *b* = outer enamel of crown; *b,* = enamel of enamel niche (the mark); *c* = root cementum; *c,* = outer crown cementum; *c,,* = enamel niche; *d* = pulp cavity; *e* = the mark.

fifteenth year by a recession of the bony wall of the alveolus and by bone apposition at the alveolar bottom, so the tooth thrusts slightly forward toward the oral cavity. The canine teeth in pigs, the incisors and posterior teeth in rodents, and the tusks of elephants are "rootless" teeth, which constantly form, grow, erupt, and shed. Anatomically speaking, "root" in this context means the enamel-free part of the tooth. The epithelial sheath grows downward without contracting; dentin and enamel are continually produced.

The permanent teeth of the diphyodont dentition develop from an epithelial germ that is tied off from the primary dental lamina at an early stage. This germ is found below the root pulp of the deciduous tooth, which is resorbed under the pressure of the replacing tooth crown (Fig. 2–4). Normally, the mortified crown of the deciduous tooth is pushed out of the alveolus by the permanent tooth. A persistent deciduous tooth occurs when the permanent crown erupts alongside the deciduous tooth and fails to cause resorption of the primary tooth root.

The molars, which are permanent teeth that erupt only once, develop from prominences (apophyses) of the primary dental lamina; strictly speaking, they are deciduous teeth that erupt later and are not replaced because no successional teeth exist to push them upward. The smaller number of deciduous posterior

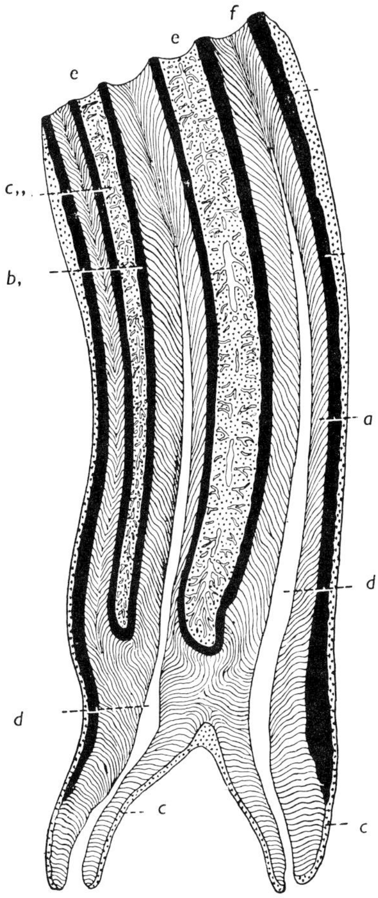

Fig. 2–3. Longitudinal section through an enamel fold posteriorly of an upper molar in horse, full size, buccal surface to the right. *a* = dentin; *b,* = enamel; *c* and *c,,* = cementum; *d* = pulp cavities of root canals; *f* = star. (From Krölling O, Grau H. Lehrbuch der Histologie und vergleichenden mikroskopischen Anatomie der Haustiere. Berlin: Paul Parey, 1960.)

teeth is adapted to the smaller jaws of young animals. A disproportionate number of teeth with respect to the length of the jaw may cause problems such as transversely lying posterior teeth in short-nosed dogs and growth disturbances of permanent premolars in early-developing young horses.

Morphologic Features (Fig. 2–5)

Dentin:

The bulk of the tooth consists of mesenchyme, formed by odontoblasts. Bone-like tissue with thin root canals is in a radial arrangement with the pulp cavity. In these root canals are prolongations of the odontoblasts (Tomes's fibers). Enamel destruction, which uncovers the dentin tubules, may cause infection of the pulp.

Enamel:

This tissue is the hardest in the body (hydroxy apatite); only 2–3% of it is organic matter. Enamel covers the crowns of cuspal enamel teeth and forms the bulk of the folding enamel teeth of herbivores. This tissue consists of

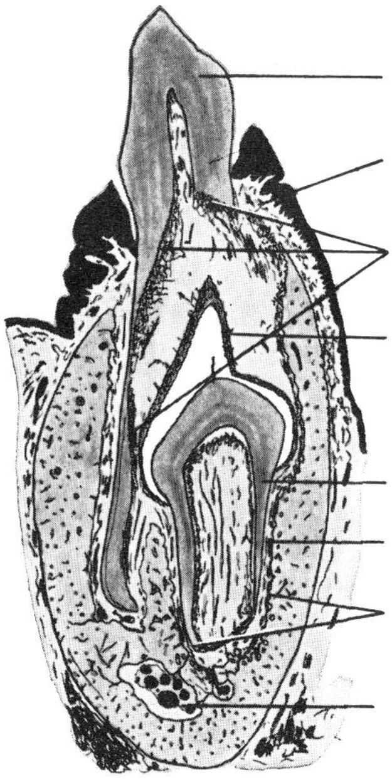

Fig. 2–4. Cross-section through a deciduous tooth that is about to be shed and a successional tooth still hidden in the alveolus of a 10-week-old cat. (From Zeitzschmann O, Krölling O. Lehrbuch der Entwicklungsgeschichte der Haustiere. Berlin: Paul Parey, 1955.)

hexagonal prisms, held together by a cementing substance, and is formed from the ectodermal enamel organ.

Cuticula dentis:

This residual substance of the outer adamantine layer is amorphously calcified and is closely connected with the cementing substance of the enamel prisms.

Dental cementum:

This substance is formed by the cementoblasts of the mesenchymal dental sac, lamellar bony tissue without dentin canals (haversian canals). It covers the enamel-free roots and is deposited between the invaginations and the enamel folds, except in the incisors and the three premolars in the mandible of horses.

Fig. 2–5. Cross-section showing the anatomic structures of the alveolus and gingiva. The dental cuticle *(a)* consists of ossified superficial epithelial enamel prisms. Enamel *(b)* covers the dentin of the crown. Dentin *(c)* which forms the bulk of the crown and root, is produced by odontoblast cells settled around the pulp cavity. From these odontoblasts, small processes are radially directed to the superficial dentin areas. A few sensory nerves are located in these channels. The pulp cavity *(d)* contains the pulp, which is composed of sensory nerves, arteries, veins, lymphatic vessels, and a primitive connective tissue. The pulp cavity is wide in young individuals and gradually narrows by apposition of new dentin. Cementum *(e)* is a thin covering of bonelike tissue found only at the roots and surrounded by the periosteum (broken lines). The Sharpey's fibers *(f)* are anchored in the cementum surface of the root and in the alveolar endosteum, thus building a strong syndesmosis. The apical foramen *(g)* at the end of each root allows free passage of the vessels and nerves through the root canal. (From Ellenberger-Baum. Handbuch der vergleichenden Anatomie der Haustiere, 18th ed. Berlin: Springer, 1943.)

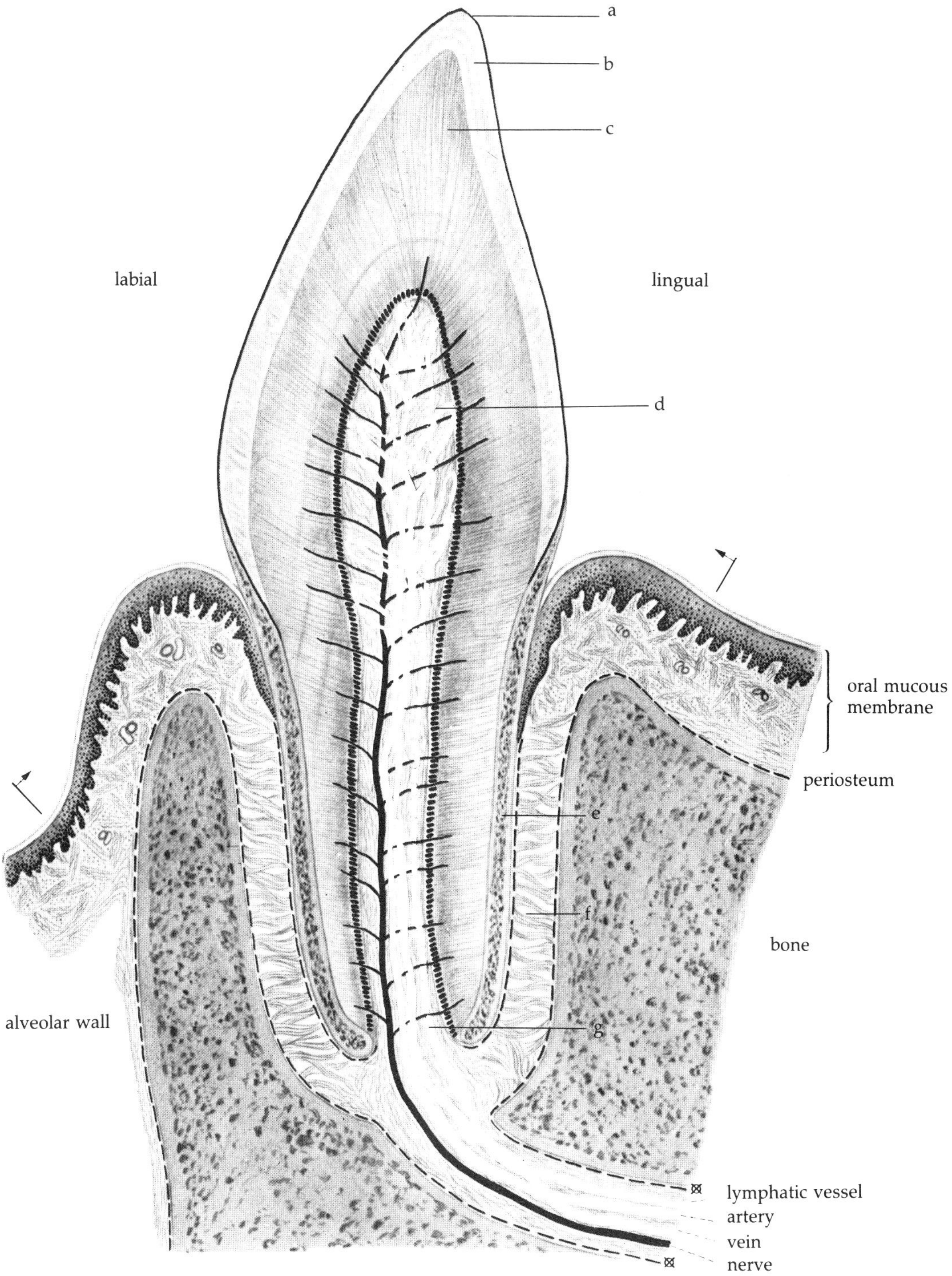
a
b
c
labial
lingual
d
oral mucous
membrane
periosteum
e
f
bone
alveolar wall
g
lymphatic vessel
artery
vein
nerve

Crown:
The crown, which comprises the bulk of the tooth, is either covered by an enamel cap or is supported by enamel folds (herbivores). It is the visible part of the tooth.

Root:
This part of the tooth contains no enamel, but is covered by cementum. The root is the invisible part of the tooth.

Tooth neck:
In cuspal enamel teeth, the neck of the tooth is the elevation with an adjacent flat groove at the transition from the crown to the root (enamel margin).

Pulp cavity:
On growing teeth, this structure is a wide cavity extending from the crown to the root apex; it is later contracted and shortened by secondary dentin toward the root canal which contains nerves and blood vessels. These nerves and blood vessels enter the pulp cavity through the apical foramen.

Dental pulp:
The pulp contains a loose, colloidal network (reticulum) of miscellaneous tissues, such as connective tissue, nerves, and lymph and blood vessels, in the developing (erupting) tooth. One layer of odontoblasts next to the dentin branches into the dental canals; these odontoblasts, together with the fine nerve endings, cause the dentin's sensitivity to temperature and pain. The odontoblasts lay down secondary dentin and thus reduce the pulp cavity in size, but at the same time, any decay of dentin may be sealed, and the pulp may be thereby protected from infection.

Alveolus:
This structure is an indentation in the jaw bone in which the root is immovably inserted. The jaw bone is connected with the root by taut fiber bundles (Sharpey's fibers), which are tightly fastened in the cementum. Thus, they form a net-like, interlacing elastic attachment of the tooth. The alveolus is surrounded by the gum tissue, which in turn is tightly attached to the bone. The gum tissue is attached to the crown of the tooth by a circular (anular) ligament, reinforced by connective tissue fibers.

ANATOMY, TOPOGRAPHY, AND NOMENCLATURE

Anatomy

Dentes decidui: deciduous dentition (incisors, canines, premolars)
Dentes permanentes: permanent dentition (successional teeth and molars)
Dentes incisivi: incisors (I)
Dentes canini: canine teeth, eye teeth, fangs (c, C)
Dentes premolares: premolars (p, P)
Dentes molares: molars (m, M)

Heterodont dentition of mammals:
Different kinds of teeth are present, such as incisors, canines, and molars.

Homodont dentition of sharks, reptiles, and fish:
All teeth are homogeneous.

Monophyodont dentition:
This form is characterized by the development of one single set of teeth, such as molars or the tusks of elephants.

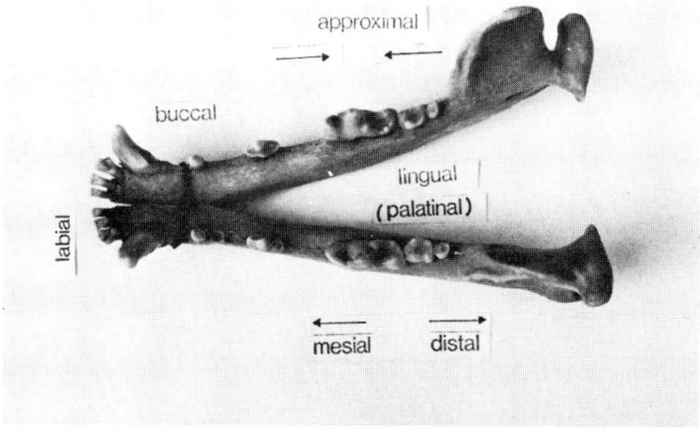

Fig. 2–6. Topographic features of the teeth.

Diphyodont dentition:
This form is characterized by development of two sets of teeth, such as in mammals.

Polyphyodont dentition:
Teeth are continually replaced, as in fish, amphibians, and reptiles.

Secodont dentition:
This form is characterized by cutting edges, lateral compression of teeth, and cusps arranged in a line, such as the premolars in carnivores and omnivores (pigs).

Bunodont dentition:
Cusps are arranged side by side to form one occlusal surface, such as the molars in humans; in cats (chiefly carnivores), only the last upper posterior tooth is nearly bunodont; in dogs (mainly carnivores), both the last upper and both last lower posterior teeth have occlusal surfaces; in herbivores, all molars and even the incisors have occlusal surfaces.

Topography (Fig. 2–6)

Mesial: surface directed toward the median line of the dental arch
Distal: surface directed away from the median line of the dental arch
Apical: relating to the apex of a tooth root
Occlusal: relating to the occlusal surface
Facies masticatoria: chewing and biting surfaces
Facies labialis: surfaces toward the lip
Facies buccalis: surfaces toward the cheek
Facies lingualis: surfaces toward the tongue
Facies contactus: contact area of two adjacent teeth

Nomenclature

Presented here are abbreviated notations for an orderly record of individual teeth for diagnostic files, statistics, and comparative data (Fig. 2–7). Tooth anatomy can be described by using capital letters for permanent teeth and lowercase letters for deciduous dentition and the words "left" and "right." Consec-

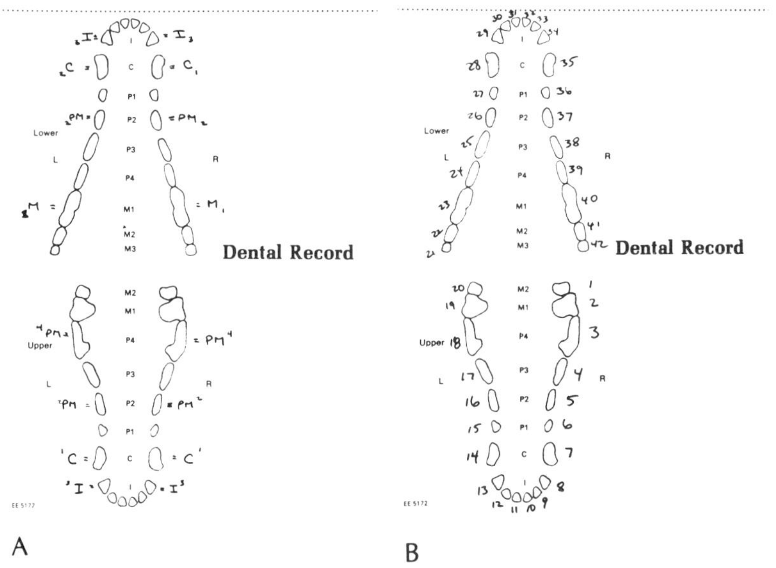

Fig. 2–7. Alternate nomenclature systems. *A*, superscripts and subscripts. Example: I^1 = maxillary first incisor right side; I_1 = mandibular first incisor left side; ^1C = maxillary left canine tooth; C_1 = mandibular right canine tooth *B*, Numeric system. Numbering of each tooth in a normal animal begins on the upper right side and ends on the lower right side. The first (No. 1) tooth is the maxillary second molar and the last tooth (No. 42) is the mandibular third molar in canine species.

utive numbering, common in human dentistry, has been introduced in veterinary dentistry, however. This method of notation starts in the median plane; the upper jaw and the lower jaw are marked by + or − symbols, or the respective numbers are provided with rectangular symbols. The graphic representation depicts the way the dentist, facing and standing over the patient, views the patient's teeth. Thus, the left half of the patient's dentition is presented on the right, and vice versa. The vertical line of the rectangular symbols and the + or − symbols always face the median line. The upper and lower jaws are divided by a horizontal line, like a fractional number.

To render the nomenclature readily accessible by computer, as well as for other practical purposes, some have recommended that the numbers 1 to 4 for permanent teeth and 5 to 8 for deciduous teeth be placed before the numbers representing the part of the jaw. Marking the parts of the jaw starts with 1 (or 5) at the upper right, and continues clockwise from the upper left to the bottom left and, finally, to bottom right. In animals with more than nine teeth in each part of the jaw, the numeral that refers to the position in the series must be a two-digit number; consequently, the new nomenclature must comprise three-digit numbers. (Table 2–1).

To avoid any misunderstanding, we recommend either Triadan's three-digit nomenclature or the anatomic nomenclature. Triadan's system offers certain advantages for technical reasons, whereas the anatomic system supplies clear, unmistakable information about the type of tooth, even in animals with a reduced dentition, such as cats and rodents (Table 2–2).

Table 2–1. Comparison of Nomenclature, Permanent Dentition in Dogs

Right											
Maxilla											
Anatomic		M 2	M 1	P 4	P 3	P 2	P 1	C	I 3	I 2	I 1
Haderup		10+	9+	8+	7+	6+	5+	4+	3+	2+	1+
Rectangular symbol		10⌋	9⌋	8⌋	7⌋	6⌋	5⌋	4⌋	3⌋	2⌋	1⌋
Triadan		110	109	108	107	106	105	104	103	102	101
Mandible Triadan	411	410	409	408	407	406	405	404	403	402	401
Rectangular symbol	11⌉	10⌉	9⌉	8⌉	7⌉	6⌉	5⌉	4⌉	3⌉	2⌉	1⌉
Haderup	11–	10–	9–	8–	7–	6–	5–	4–	3–	2–	1–
Anatomic	M 3	M 2	M 1	P 4	P 3	P 2	P 1	C	I 3	I 2	I 1

Left											
Maxilla											
Anatomic	I 1	I 2	I 3	C	P 1	P 2	P 3	P 4	M 1	M 2	
Haderup	+1	+2	+3	+4	+5	+6	+7	+8	+9	+10	
Rectangular symbol	⌊1	⌊2	⌊3	⌊4	⌊5	⌊6	⌊7	⌊8	⌊9	⌊10	
Triadan	201	202	203	204	205	206	207	208	209	210	
Mandible Triadan	301	302	303	304	305	306	307	308	309	310	311
Rectangular symbol	⌈1	⌈2	⌈3	⌈4	⌈5	⌈6	⌈7	⌈8	⌈9	⌈10	⌈11
Haderup	–1	–2	–3	–4	–5	–6	–7	–8	–9	–10	–11
Anatomic	I 1	I 2	I 3	C	P 1	P 2	P 3	P 4	M 1	M 2	M 3

M = Molar; P = premolar; C = canine; I = incisor

Table 2–2. Nomenclature of Deciduous Dentition

Right							*Left*						
Pd 3	Pd 2	Pd 1	Cd	Id 3	Id 2	Id 1	Id 1	Id 2	Id 3	Cd	Pd 1	Pd 2	Pd 3
p 3	p 2	p 1	c	i 3	i 2	i 1	i 1	i 2	i 3	c	p 1	p 2	p 3
507	506	505	504	503	502	501	601	602	603	604	605	606	607
807	806	805	804	803	802	801	701	702	703	704	705	706	707

P, p = Premolar; C, c = canine; I, i = incisor; d = deciduous

FUNCTIONING OF THE MASTICATORY SYSTEM

The main function of the temporal muscle in carnivores is biting and seizing food. The masticatory force depends on the length and strength of the mandible (lever of the first class). The masseter and pterygoid muscles are responsible for mastication in herbivores. The innervation of the masticatory muscles is through the branches of the mandibular nerve, which is the only motor branch of the trigeminal nerve.

Carnivores

The temporal muscle covers the temporal fossa. Origin: temporal fossa; attachment: coronoid process of the mandible.

The deep masseter muscle is stronger than the intermediate and superficial masseter muscles. Origin: maxillary tuber, malar arch; attachment: ramus of the mandible.

The stronger medial pterygoid muscle covers the lateral pterygoid muscle to the pharynx. Origin: lateral to the pterygoid, sphenoid bone wing; attachment: ramus of the mandible.

Functioning of Teeth

Incisors: biting and gnawing, hygiene.

Canines: seizing and tearing of food.

Molars: shearing of soft tissue and bones. In dogs, the back molars have occlusal surfaces with fissures and cusps.

The masticatory force in the molar zone may reach 3000 kg/cm^2, but it differs according to breed, age, sex, and usual food. All around dogs trained as watch dogs may produce forces of 500 kg/cm^2 in the canine zone.

Herbivores

The masseter muscle is strong, broad, and sinewy. Origin: along the zygomatic arch; attachment: ramus of the mandible.

The pterygoid muscle is also strong, particularly the medial pterygoid muscle. The origin and attachment are the same as in carnivores. The contraction of the lateral pterygoid muscle moves the mandible toward the maxilla. The masseter, temporal, and pterygoid muscles pull the mandible away from the maxilla.

The temporalis muscle is weaker than the pterygoid muscles. The temporomandibular joint of herbivores is in a transverse position and is slightly vaulted, thus allowing lateral movement.

The incisors tear off grass and bark and, together with the lips, take in feed, which is then ground by the molars.

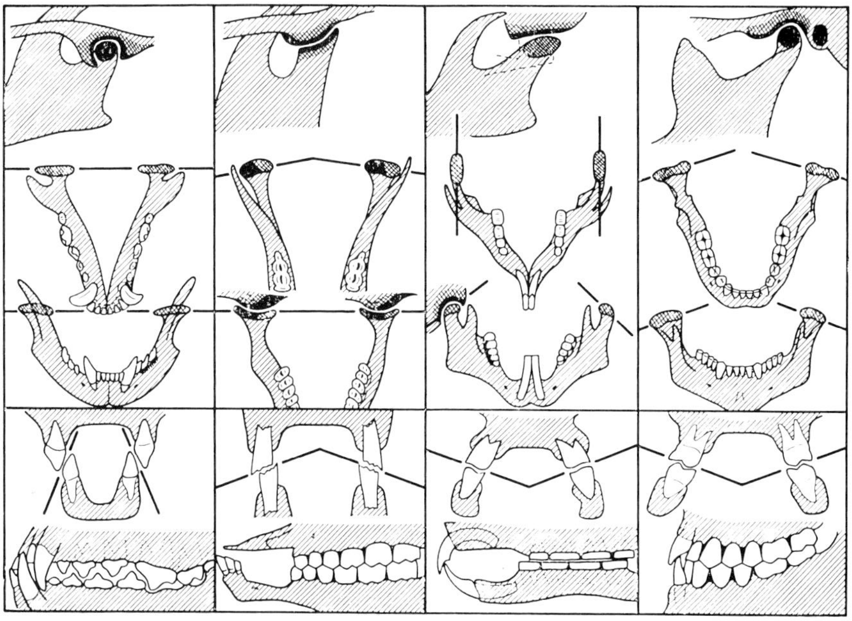

Fig. 2–8. Proportional schematic representation of temporomandibular joints and teeth in animals and in man. Carnivores: tearing of food by incisors and canines; maxillary occlusal surfaces cover the mandibular antagonists vestibularly; temporomandibular joints are hinged. Ruminants: mincing of food by lateral mandibular movements. Rodents: mastication mainly by forward and backward movements of the mandible; the joints slide sled-like in grooved glenoid cavities in some species. Primates: the temporomandibular joints of monkeys are similar to those in humans; they can perform mandibular movements typical of those of carnivores, ruminants, and rodents. (From Joest E. Handbuch der speziellen pathologischen Anatomie der Haustiere, 3rd ed (vol 5). Berlin: Paul Parey, 1967.)

Rodents

The rodent's strongest masticatory muscle is the temporal muscle, which retracts the mandible and is an antagonist to the pterygoid muscles.

The masseter muscle functions in much the same way as in other domestic animals.

The bilateral tension of the pterygoid muscle causes a forward movement of the mandible. The temporomandibular joint is on a longitudinal groove, which allows a forward-and-backward sliding movement. To some extent, a rotary movement is possible, although it is absent in rabbits. The incisors mince the feed or its hard shell, and the molars grind it.

Pigs

The seizing and tearing of food is done with the middle teeth of the jaw, as in carnivores. Chewing takes place farther back toward the throat.

Primates

The chewing muscles and the temporomandibular joint are arranged as in humans; the mandible is movable in every direction.

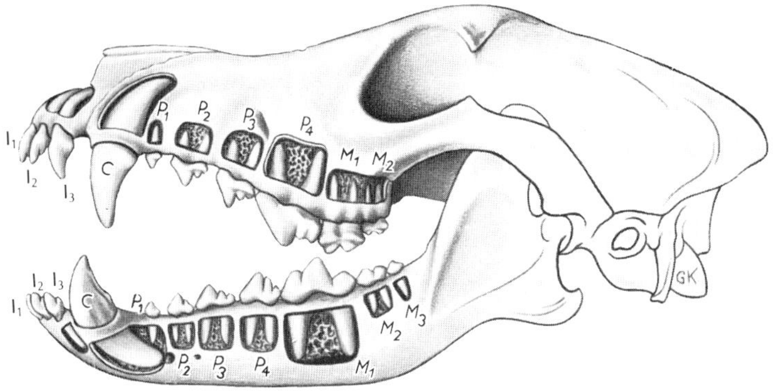

Fig. 2–9. Permanent, normal dentition of an 8-month-old sheep dog. Sections removed to show roots; P4 in the maxilla and M1 in the mandible are sectorial teeth. (From Nickel R, Schummer A, Seiferle E. Lehrbuch der Anatomie der Haustiere, 4th ed (vol 2). Berlin: Paul Parey, 1979.)

DENTITION OF DIFFERENT DOMESTIC ANIMALS (Fig. 2–8)

The anatomic method of nomenclature distinguishes the types of teeth in each half of the upper and lower jaws. Deciduous teeth are represented as lowercase letters or as capital letters with an additional "d" (for deciduous); permanent teeth and replacement teeth are represented by capital letters. A phylogenetically complete dental formula, found only in the wild boar and the mole, is as follows:

$$\frac{3I \quad 1C \quad 4P \quad 3M}{3I \quad 1C \quad 4P \quad 3M} = 44$$

Dogs (Fig. 2–9 and Table 2–3)

Deciduous dentition

$$\frac{3i \quad 1c \quad 3p}{3i \quad 1c \quad 3p} = 28$$

Permanent dentition

$$\frac{3I \quad 1C \quad 4P \quad 2M}{3I \quad 1C \quad 4P \quad 3M} = 42$$

Carnivores have cuspal enamel teeth. The crowns of I1 and I2 in the maxilla are trilobate; the crown of maxillary I3 is conical; the crowns of I1 to I3 in the mandible are bilobate. In the normal dentition of dolichocephalic breeds, such as the Alsatian, the lower canine tooth fits into the diastema of I3 and C in the maxilla when the mouth is closed. The maxillary premolars fit into the spaces between the mandibular premolars.

The brachycephalic breeds, such as the boxer, have larger spaces between the mandibular premolars than do other breeds. The upper canine tooth is about the right size to fit into the space between the mandibular P2 and P3 when the mouth is closed. The shortened upper maxilla should have all 20 teeth, which grow at an angle because of the lack of space.

In a normal dentition, the mandible is usually narrower and longer than the maxilla (anisognathous); therefore, the lower incisors and molars are angled inward in relation to the maxillary teeth (shear mouth). An exception are the bunodont configurations of both the maxillary and the mandibular M1 and M2, which come into direct contact with each other (Table 2–3).

Table 2–3. Eruption and Change of Teeth in Dogs

Teeth		*Age erupted*	*Teeth*		*Age changed*
Id	$\frac{1}{1}$		I	$\frac{1}{1}$	
Id	$\frac{2}{2}$	4–6 weeks	I	$\frac{2}{2}$	3–5 months
Id	$\frac{3}{3}$		I	$\frac{3}{3}$	
Cd	$\frac{1}{1}$	3–5 weeks	C	$\frac{1}{1}$	5–7 months
Pd	$\frac{1}{1}$	4–5 months			no change
Pd	$\frac{2}{2}$		P	$\frac{2}{2}$	
Pd	$\frac{3}{3}$	5–6 weeks	P	$\frac{3}{3}$	5–6 months
Pd	$\frac{4}{4}$		P	$\frac{4}{4}$	
M	$\frac{1}{1}$	4–5 months			
M	$\frac{2}{2}$	5–6 months			
M	$\frac{-}{3}$	6–7 months			

I = Incisor; C = canine; P = premolar; M = molar; d = deciduous
(From Nickel R, Schummer A, Seiferle E. Lehrbuch der Anatomie der Haustiere, 4th ed (vol 2). Berlin: Paul Parey, 1979.)

The incisors, canines, and first premolars of both jaws, as well as the third molar of the mandible, are single rooted. P2 and P3 in the maxilla as well as P2 to P4 and M1 and M2 in the mandible have two roots. P4, M1, and M2 in the maxilla have three roots.

P1 erupts as a permanent tooth in both the maxilla and the mandible; in a way, these premolars are persistent deciduous teeth.

Shearing teeth:

$$\frac{\text{p3}}{\text{p4}} \text{ and } \frac{\text{P4}}{\text{M1}}$$

In this zone, the greatest force is exerted by the masticatory muscles because of favorable leverage. The dog possesses a fully functional dentition at an early age, although the schedules of eruption and change of teeth depend on the breed and on the individual dog.

Cats (Figs. 2–10 and 2–11 and Table 2–4)

Deciduous dentition

$$\frac{\text{3i 1c 3p}}{\text{3i 1c 2p}} = 26$$

Permanent dentition

$$\frac{\text{3I 1C 3P 1M}}{\text{3I 1C 2P 1M}} = 30$$

Proportionate with its short jaw bones, the cat's dentition is reduced in the

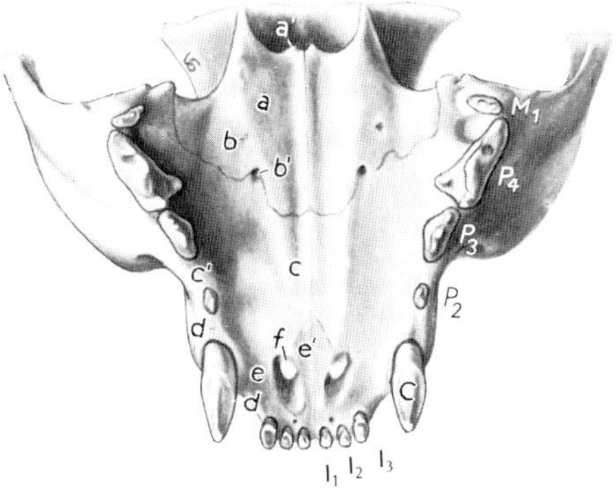

Fig. 2–10. The maxillary arch of a 7-month-old cat. *I1 to 3*: dentes incisivi; *C*: dens caninus; *P2* to 4: dentes premolares; *M1*: dens molaris; *a*: pars horizontalis of the os palatinum with *a'* of the spina nasalis caudalis; *b*: foramen palatinum majus; *c*: processus palatinus; *c'*: processus alveolaris of the maxilla; *d*: diastema; *e* and *e'*: processus palatinus of the os incisivum; *f*: fissura palatina. (From Nickel R, Schummer A, Seiferle E. Lehrbuch der Anatomie der Haustiere, 5th ed (vol 2). Berlin: Paul Parey, 1982.)

premolar and molar zones. The first two premolars in the mandible of dogs are absent in cats. P2 and M1 in the maxilla are proportionately small, when compared with a dog's dentition.

The molars have no occlusal surfaces; they are therefore secodont. The mandibular canine tooth fits into the diastema of I3 and C in the maxilla when the mouth is closed. The teeth in the narrower mandible are in centric occlusion with those in the maxilla and are angled inward in relation to them (shear mouth).

The incisors and canines are single rooted; P3, P4, and M1 in the mandible are doubled rooted. In the maxilla, P2 has one root, P3 and M1 have two roots, and P4 has three roots.

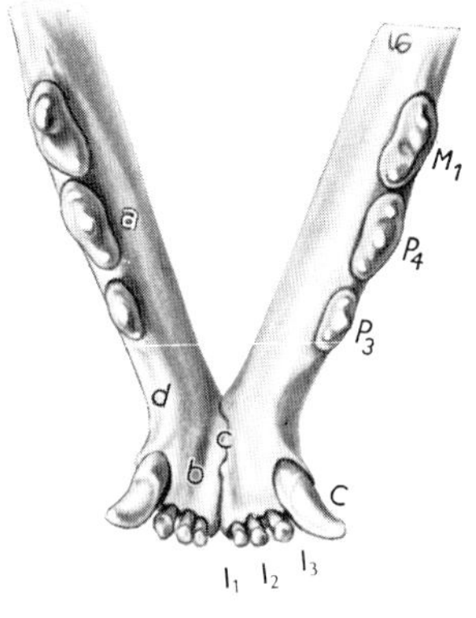

Fig. 2–11. The mandibular arch of a 7-month-old cat. *I1 to 3*: dentes incisivi; *C*: dens caninus; *P3* and *P4*: dentes premolares; *a*: pars molaris; *b*: pars incisiva mandibulae; *c*: symphysis mandibulae; *d*: diastema. (From Nickel R, Schummer A, Seiferle E. Lehrbuch der Anatomie der Haustiere, 5th ed (vol 2). Berlin: Paul Parey, 1982.)

Table 2–4. Eruption and Change of Teeth in Cats

Teeth	*Age erupted*	*Teeth*	*Age changed*
Id $\frac{1}{1}$		I $\frac{1}{1}$	
Id $\frac{2}{2}$	3–4 weeks	I $\frac{2}{2}$	3½–5½ months
Id $\frac{3}{3}$		I $\frac{3}{3}$	
Cd $\frac{1}{1}$		C $\frac{1}{1}$	5½–6½ months
Pd $\frac{2}{}$		P $\frac{2}{}$	
Pd $\frac{3}{3}$	5–6 weeks	P $\frac{3}{3}$	4–5 months
Pd $\frac{4}{4}$		P $\frac{4}{4}$	
M $\frac{1}{1}$			

I = Incisor; C = canine; P = premolar; M = molar; d = deciduous
(From Nickel R, Schummer A, Seiferle E. Lehrbuch der Anatomie der Haustiere, 4th ed (vol 2). Berlin: Paul Parey, 1979.)

Shearing teeth:

$$\frac{P4}{M1}$$

Horses (Fig. 2–12 and Table 2–5)

Deciduous dentition

$$\frac{3i \quad 1c \quad 3p}{3i \quad 1c \quad 3p} = 28$$

Permanent dentition

$$\frac{3I \quad 1C \quad 3(4)P \quad 3M}{3I \quad 1C \quad 3 \quad P \quad 3M} = 40\ (42)$$

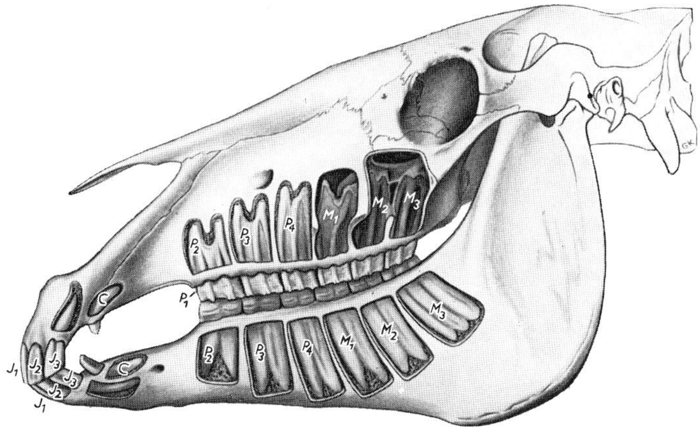

Fig. 2–12. Permanent dentition of an 8-year-old gelding. Sections removed to show roots. (From Nickel R, Schummer A, Seiferle E. Lehrbuch der Anatomie der Haustiere, 5th ed (vol 2). Berlin: Paul Parey, 1982.) (*Note:* Teeth with label "J" indicate incisors.)

Table 2–5. Eruption and Change of Teeth in Horses

Teeth		*Age erupted*	*Teeth*		*Age changed*
Id	$\frac{1}{1}$	prenatally and during the first days after birth	I	$\frac{1}{1}$	2½–3 years
Id	$\frac{2}{2}$	3–4 weeks, occasionally up to 8 weeks	I	$\frac{2}{2}$	3½–4 years
Id	$\frac{3}{3}$	5–9 months	I	$\frac{3}{3}$	4½–5 years
Cd	$\frac{1}{1}$	Eruption is rare	C	$\frac{1}{1}$	4–5 years
Pd	$\frac{2}{2}$		P	$\frac{2}{2}$	2½ years
Pd	$\frac{3}{3}$	prenatally or in the first week after birth	P	$\frac{3}{3}$	2½ years
Pd	$\frac{4}{4}$		P	$\frac{4}{4}$	3½ years
M	$\frac{1}{1}$	6–9 months, rarely up to 14 months			
M	$\frac{2}{2}$	2–2½ years			
M	$\frac{3}{3}$	3½–4½ years			

I = Incisor; C = canine; P = premolar; M = molar; d = deciduous

(From Nickel R, Schummer A, Seiferle E. Lehrbuch der Anatomie der Haustiere, 4th ed (vol 2). Berlin: Paul Parey, 1979.)

The incisors, premolars, and molars have an enamel fold structure. The crown of the canine tooth is cuspal.

Incisors

Incisor I1 is the central incisor, I2 is the lateral incisor, and I3 is the corner incisor. These teeth are arranged in a dental arch. The extra-alveolar part of the tooth is sharply curved; in young horses, the occlusal surfaces do not contact each other (edge-to-edge occlusion). When these teeth become abraded, at the rate of about 2 mm per year, the straighter bulk of the tooth is pushed out of the jaw. Temporarily, the occlusal surfaces are unable to contact each other; the first and second notches, which are essential for estimating the animal's age develop at the still strongly curved maxillary canines. Eventually, the growing, straighter parts of teeth form the angled dentition. The occlusal surfaces in the young horse have a vertically oval cross-section that, toward the root, becomes round, triangular, and horizontally oval. This change is also essential when estimating the animal's age.

The occlusal enamel cup or infundibulum is 2 mm deep in the upper incisor and 6 mm deep in the lower incisor. In the labial direction, the end of the pulp cavity is gradually filled by secondary dentin, and in older animals becomes visible as a dental star caused by the deposition of hemoglobin fragments.

The deciduous incisors have a shovel-shaped crown and a distinct dental neck (collum dentis). These incisors are small and whiter than the successional teeth. The labial surface has 2 longitudinal grooves; the enamel cup is 4-mm deep (Table 2–5).

Canines

The upper and lower canines in both sexes are deciduous teeth that do not erupt, although they are sometimes found in mares as permanent teeth that rarely erupt.

Premolars and Molars

Between the canines and premolars is the toothless interalveolar margin, which is the interarch distance. The adjacent rudimentary p1 (wolf tooth or dens angularis) rarely erupts in the maxilla. If it does, it is shed early and is not replaced. Clinically significant lesions may be caused in this zone by the snaffle.

The molar region usually begins with the mesial p2/P2; p4/P4 is next to M1.

In horses, the P4 next to the M1 is frequently called P1; thus, the most mesial tooth becomes P3. This numbering method takes into account the existence of an occasional P4 (the adjacent rudimentary P1) and obviates the need to term the first tooth in the molar region P2, which initially seems illogical.

The deciduous premolars are more delicate than the successional premolars, although they are otherwise similar to them.

The upper posterior teeth have a square cross-section, and their crowns have compact enamel cups, similar to those of the incisors, that are filled with cementum. Because of the stronger abrasion of cementum and dentin, two map-like areas are formed at the harder enamel margins. The outside of the tooth body is partly covered by cementum, which also fills the deep enamel folds. Three short roots are formed in fully grown animals 6 to 7 years old.

The lower posterior teeth are slender and have a rectangular cross-section. Their crowns have no enamel cups; therefore, the deep enamel folds are open at the crown and root and are filled by dentin. The outer surfaces of the enamel folds are covered by cementum, thereby sealing the grooves. The lower molars form two root stumps.

The molars in horses are anisognathous; the molar zone of the mandibular dental arch is narrower than the corresponding part of the maxillary dental arch. The temporomandibular joint of the herbivore allows lateral movements as well as central occlusion; however, the molars of the mandible are always on the lingual side of the maxillary molars. Therefore, clinically significant sharp tooth apexes of the upper molars are found on the buccal side, whereas those of the lower molars are found on the lingual side.

Ruminants (Fig. 2–13 and Table 2–6)

Deciduous dentition

$$\frac{0i \quad 0c \quad 3p}{3i \quad 1c \quad 3p} = 20$$

Permanent dentition

$$\frac{0I \quad 0C \quad 3P \quad 3M}{3I \quad 1C \quad 3P \quad 3M} = 32$$

No maxillary incisors or canine teeth are present, but ontogenetic evidence

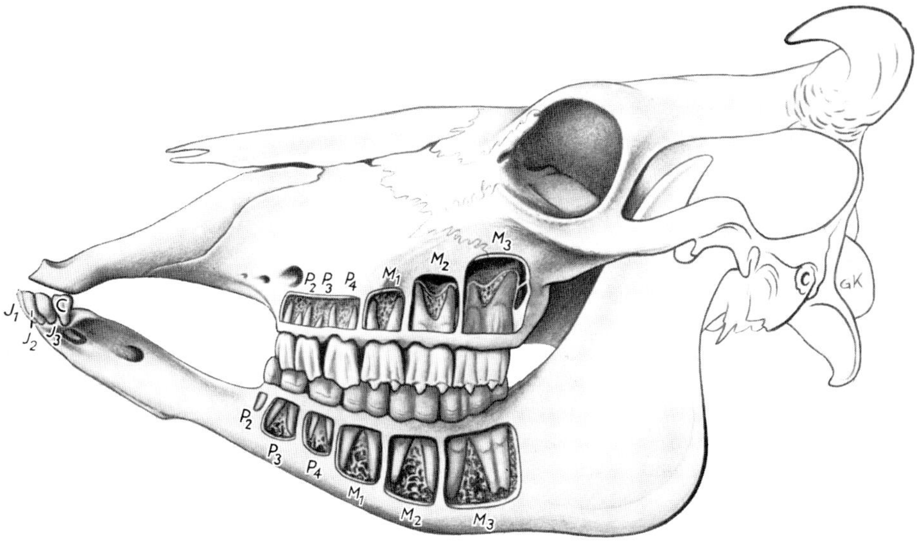

Fig. 2–13. Permanent dentition of an 8-year-old cow. Sections removed to show roots. (From Nickel R, Schummer A, Seiferle E. Lehrbuch der Anatomie der Haustiere, 4th ed (vol 2). Berlin: Paul Parey, 1979.) (*Note:* Teeth with label "J" indicate incisors.)

Table 2–6. Eruption and Change of Teeth in Cattle

Teeth		*Age erupted*	*Teeth*		*Age changed*
Id	$\frac{-}{1}$	before birth	I	$\frac{-}{1}$	14–25 months
Id	$\frac{-}{2}$	before birth	I	$\frac{-}{2}$	17–33 months
Id	$\frac{-}{3}$	before birth up to 2–6 days	I	$\frac{-}{3}$	22–40 months
Cd		before birth up to 2–14 days	C		32–42 months
Pd	$\frac{2}{2}$	before birth up to 14–21 days	P	$\frac{2}{2}$	24–28 months
Pd	$\frac{3}{3}$	before birth up to 14–21 days	P	$\frac{3}{3}$	24–30 months
Pd	$\frac{4}{4}$	before birth up to 14–21 days	P	$\frac{4}{4}$	28–34 months
M	$\frac{1}{1}$	5–6 months			
M	$\frac{2}{2}$	15–18 months			
M	$\frac{3}{3}$	24–28 months			

I = Incisor; C = canine; P = premolar; M = molar; d = deciduous
(From Nickel R, Schummer A, Seiferle E. Lehrbuch der Anatomie der Haustiere, 4th ed (vol 2). Berlin: Paul Parey, 1979.)

Table 2–7. Eruption and Change of Teeth in Sheep

Teeth		*Age erupted*	*Teeth*		*Age changed*
Id	$\overline{1}$	before birth up to 8 days	I	$\overline{1}$	12–18 months
Id	$\overline{2}$	before birth	I	$\overline{2}$	21–24 months
Id	$\overline{3}$	before birth	I	$\overline{3}$	27–36 months
Cd		at birth up to 8 days	C		36–48 months
Pd	$\frac{2}{2}$	before birth up to 4 weeks	P	$\frac{2}{2}$	21–24 months
Pd	$\frac{3}{3}$	before birth up to 4 weeks	P	$\frac{3}{3}$	21–24 months
Pd	$\frac{4}{4}$	before birth up to 4 weeks	P	$\frac{4}{4}$	21–24 months
M	$\frac{1}{1}$	3 months			
M	$\frac{2}{2}$	9 months			
M	$\frac{3}{3}$	18 months			

I = Incisor; C = canine; P = premolar; M = molar; d = deciduous
(From Nickel R, Schummer A, Seiferle E. Lehrbuch der Anatomie der Haustiere, 4th ed (vol 2). Berlin: Paul Parey, 1979.)

proves that they once existed in both cattle and sheep. In the place of these teeth, the cornified dental plate serves as a frictional surface for the mandibular incisors.

The three mandibular incisors and the modified canine tooth that erupts close to them form the incisor arch. The crowns are shovel shaped, the dental necks are clearly marked, and the roots are short, round, and curved. Thus, the incisors are not firmly anchored and are often shed in older animals. In young animals, the crowns of the permanent incisors overlap like roofing tiles; not until the jaw grows do they form a complete dental arch. The incisors and modified canines are termed the central incisor, inner lateral incisor, and outer lateral incisor (or corner incisor) (Table 2–7).

Premolars and Molars

The molar region starts with P2; the teeth are progressively stronger distally (aborally). Nearly all of them have enamel folds and consist of one to three prism-like elements with an enamel cup on each crown. Enamel cups and outer folds are filled with cementum. Deciduous p2 and p3 in the mandible each consist of one prism-like element without an enamel cup; p3 and p4 have two elements with two enamel cups. The mandibular posterior teeth are narrow and rectangular; the maxillary posterior teeth are nearly square in cross-section. The permanent mandibular premolars have two roots. P2 has a conical enamel cusp, P3 and P4 are flattened and have, in most cases, no enamel cusp. The permanent maxillary premolars have three roots; each has a sickle-shaped cup on the wide occlusal surface.

Table 2–8. Eruption and Change of Teeth in Goats

Teeth	*Age erupted*	*Teeth*	*Age changed*
Id $\frac{-}{1}$	at birth	I $\frac{-}{1}$	15 months
Id $\frac{-}{2}$	at birth	I $\frac{-}{2}$	21 months
Id $\frac{-}{3}$	at birth	I $\frac{-}{3}$	27 months
Cd	1–3 weeks	C	36 months
Pd $\frac{2}{2}$	3 months	P $\frac{2}{2}$	17–20 months
Pd $\frac{3}{3}$	3 months	P $\frac{3}{3}$	17–20 months
Pd $\frac{4}{4}$	3 months	P $\frac{4}{4}$	17–20 months
M $\frac{1}{1}$	5–6 months		
M $\frac{2}{2}$	8–10 months		
M $\frac{3}{3}$	18–24 months		

I = Incisor; C = canine; P = premolar; M = molar; d = deciduous
(From Nickel R, Schummer A, Seiferle E. Lehrbuch der Anatomie der Haustiere, 4th ed (vol 2). Berlin: Paul Parey, 1979.)

The mandibular molars are narrow and have two roots. M1 and M2 consist of two prism-like elements each; M3 consists of three such elements; they have two cups each (Table 2–8). The maxillary molars have three roots and consist of two elements each. Each tooth has two enamel cups on the occlusal surface.

The mandibular rami in cattle are much closer to each other than are the opposing sides of the maxillary molar region (anisognathous). The temporomandibular joint allows lateral grinding occlusion, so only the teeth of either half of the jaw are fully in contact at one time. The dentition of sheep and goats is similar to that in cattle (see Tables 2–7 and 2–8). The occlusal surface is inclined, and a sharp ridge thereby develops. In the maxilla, this ridge is on the buccal side. In the mandible, it is on the lingual side.

Pigs (Fig. 2–14 and Table 2–9)

Deciduous dentition

$$\frac{3i \quad 1c \quad 3p}{3i \quad 1c \quad 3p} = 28$$

Permanent dentition

$$\frac{3I \quad 1C \quad 4P \quad 3M}{3I \quad 1C \quad 4P \quad 3M} = 44$$

The pig has the most complete dentition of all domestic mammals; even P1 is regularly developed. The teeth have enamel cusps; particularly worth mentioning is the rootless canine tooth, which continues to grow throughout the animal's life.

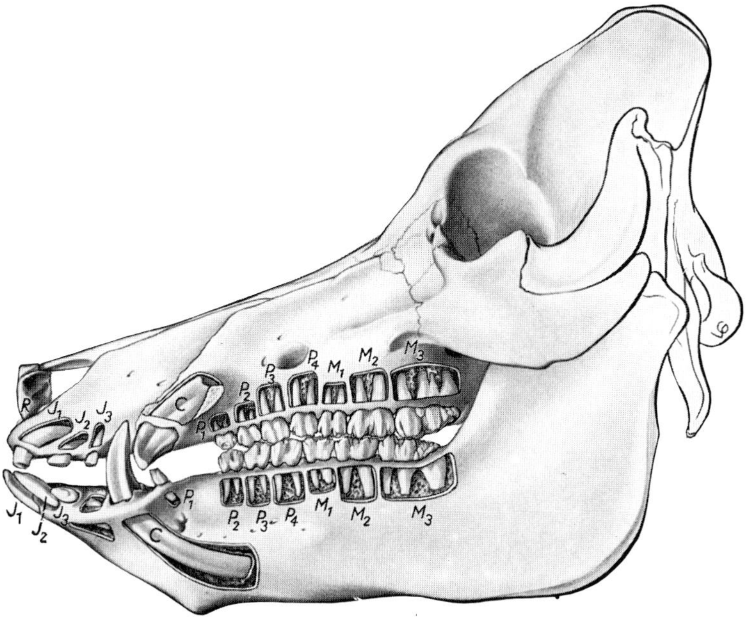

Fig. 2–14. Permanent dentition of a 2-year-old boar. Sections removed to show roots. (From Nickel R, Schummer A, Seiferle E. Lehrbuch der Anatomie der Haustiere, 4th ed (vol 2). Berlin: Paul Parey, 1979.) (*Note:* Teeth with label "J" indicate incisors.)

Incisors

I1 and I2 in the mandible are straight and chisel shaped, with a strong, square root. I3 is smaller than I1 and I2. Both maxillary I1 teeth are arched and curved toward the center line; they exert frictional force on the mandibular I1 and I2. The maxillary I3 is widely separated distally from I1 and I2 and has no mandibular antagonist. Deciduous and permanent teeth have similar arrangements.

Canines

The mandibular canine tooth (tusk, fang) is larger than its antagonist and is firmly and deeply set in its socket. It is triangular and curved. Its apex is kept sharp by abrasion on the aboral maxillary canine. The maxillary canine is shorter and grows upward in a lateral curve. The canines in the sow are not as strong as those in the boar.

Premolars

The deciduous premolars (p1) in both the maxilla and mandible frequently fail to erupt. P1, therefore, erupts as a permanent tooth. The permanent premolars increase in size distally. The crowns of the mandibular P2 to P4 are laterally compressed and form a sharp edge. Because of its ridge-like crown, P1 in the maxilla has a cutting function.

P1 in the mandible is located directly behind the canine tooth; the interdental space separates it from P2. In the mandible, P2 exerts frictional force on P1 in the maxilla; P1 and P2 have two roots each, P3 has two or three roots, and P4 has three roots. In the maxilla, P1 has two roots, P2 and P3 have three roots,

Table 2–9. Eruption and Change of Teeth in Pigs

Teeth		*Age erupted*	*Teeth*		*Age changed*
Id	$\frac{1}{1}$	1–3 weeks 4–14 days	I	$\frac{1}{1}$	12–17 months
Id	$\frac{2}{2}$	10–14 weeks 8–12 weeks	I	$\frac{2}{2}$	17–18 months
Id	$\frac{3}{3}$	prenatal	I	$\frac{3}{3}$	8–12 months
Cd	$\frac{1}{1}$	prenatal	C	$\frac{1}{1}$	8–12 months
Pd	$\frac{1}{1}$	3½–6½ months			
Pd	$\frac{2}{2}$	7–10 weeks	P	$\frac{2}{2}$	12–16 months
Pd	$\frac{3}{3}$	1–3 weeks 1–5 weeks	P	$\frac{3}{3}$	12–16 months
Pd	$\frac{4}{4}$	1–4 weeks 2–7 weeks	P	$\frac{4}{4}$	12–16 months
M	$\frac{1}{1}$	4–6 months			
M	$\frac{2}{2}$	7–13 months			
M	$\frac{3}{3}$	17–22 months			

I = Incisor; C = canine; P = premolar; M = molar; d = deciduous
(From Nickel R, Schummer A, Seiferle E. Lehrbuch der Anatomie der Haustiere, 4th ed (vol 2). Berlin: Paul Parey, 1979.)

and P4 has four or five roots. P3 and P4 develop a wide occlusal surface by abrading the tricuspid crowns.

Molars

Molars also become stronger distally. Their occlusal surfaces have four to six major cusps and a number of minor cusps. M1 and M2 in the mandible have four roots each; M3 has six roots. All molars in the maxilla have six roots each and are firmly anchored in the jaw bone.

The pig's dentition is, in spite of central occlusion, isognathous; only the premolars in the maxilla are separated and overlap the antagonists in shear fashion.

Rodents (Guinea Pig, Mouse, Rat, Hamster, Squirrel, but not Hare and Rabbit)

The incisors are covered by enamel only labially and laterally. The lingual sides consist of softer dentin and some cementum, which allows stronger abrasion. In this way, a sharp, chisel-shaped labial edge develops. The intra-alveolar dental bulk extends distally as far as the posterior teeth. The incisors, and frequently the posterior teeth, have no anatomic roots; they grow throughout the animal's life. Rodents have a monophyodont dentition (no deciduous teeth). No canine teeth are present. Between the incisors and the premolars is a wide, toothless ridge. The posterior teeth have deep fissures on their lingual sides. Those in the maxilla have shallow fissures on their buccal sides as well. They lie transversely and have enamel edges on their occlusal surfaces. The jaw moves forward and backward.

Guinea Pigs

$$\frac{1I \quad 0C \quad 1P \quad 3M}{1I \quad 0C \quad 1P \quad 3M} = 20$$

The frictional surfaces of the mandibular posterior teeth are bucally inclined; those in the maxilla are lingually inclined. This feature accounts for the bridge-like overgrowth of the tongue in older animals.

Mice and Rats

$$\frac{1I \quad 0C \quad 0P \quad 3M}{1I \quad 0C \quad 0P \quad 3M} = 16$$

The rat's incisors grow about 2 to 3 mm per week.

Squirrels

$$\frac{1I \quad 0C \quad 2(1)P \quad 3M}{1I \quad 0C \quad 1\ \ P \quad 3M} = 22$$

The first premolar is small or may be missing. The incisors are usually pigmented.

Hares and Rabbits

$$\frac{2I \quad 0C \quad 3P \quad 3M}{1I \quad 0C \quad 2P \quad 3M} = 28$$

Two incisors are present in either half of the maxilla. I1 is large and is visible from the front. I2 is small, pin-shaped, and is found behind I1. A rudimentary third incisor is shed shortly after birth. Unlike in other rodents, the incisors are completely covered by dentin. Therefore, they wear away regularly. The masticatory movement is lateral because the mandibular fossa is horizontally oval. The incisors and premolars have no anatomic roots; they grow throughout the animal's life. The incisors grow as much as 11 to 12 cm per year. The posterior teeth have deep lateral enamel folds and lie transversely; M3 is tiny. Corner incisors are not present.

ESTIMATION OF AN ANIMAL'S AGE BY TOOTH ABRASION

Eruption and change of teeth are presented in tabular form in the previous section of this chapter. Early-developing breeds of horses change about 2 months earlier than those given in the table. Exact statements of age based on wear of teeth are only possible in horses and, within limits, in cattle. In other animals, variations according to breed, individual disposition, nature of food, working capacity, and individual habit overcomplicate the estimation process.

Table 2–10. Ages at which Changes Occur in the Horse's Permanent Teeth

Maxilla	*I 1*	*I 2*	*I 3*	*C*
	(years)	(years)	(years)	
Inverted oval frictional surface	27	28	29	
Triangular frictional surface	21	22	23	
Dental star	16	17	18	
Round frictional surface	15	16	17	
Disappearance of infundibulum (mark)	9	10	11	
In friction	3	4	5	
Change of teeth	2½	3½	4½	(3–6)
Mandible				
Change of teeth	2½	3½	4½	(3–6)
In friction	3	4	5	
Infundibulum (mark) disappeared	6	7	8	
Round frictional surface	12	13	14	
Dental star	13	14	15	
Triangular friction surface	18	19	20	
Inverted oval frictional surface	24	25	26	

Horses

Disappearance of the Infundibulum

i1	i2	i3
1 year	1–1½ years	2 years

In both the maxilla and the mandible, abrasion occurs almost simultaneously. The change of deciduous teeth in the maxilla takes place 2 to 8 months earlier than in the mandible (Table 2–10).

Galvayne's groove appears on the gingival margin of the maxillary I3 at the age of 10 years, on the upper half of the tooth at 15 years, and on the occlusal surface at 20 years. The end of the groove appears on the gingival margin at 20 years, on the lower half of the tooth at 25 years, and on the occlusal surface at 30 years. By x-ray examination, the time of change and eruption of posterior teeth may be employed for estimating the animal's age.

Cows

At first, the deciduous incisors are arranged like roofing tiles; the dental arch begins to expand about a month after birth. In 6 months, half the occlusal surface is in friction; in a year, the whole occlusal surface of the incisors is in friction. The permanent incisors are also arranged like roofing tiles.

The frictional surfaces of I1 and I2 are horizontally oval at the age of 5 to 7 years; they are indented between 7 and 9 years of age, round between years 9 and 11, and vertically oval between years 11 and 13. Later, only tooth stumps remain.

Bibliography: 5, 11, 14, 16, 19, 22, 27, 28, 30, 32, 33, 36, 55, 57, 63, 65

3

Technology of Dentistry

INSTRUMENTS

Dogs and Cats

Extraction

Veterinary Oral Surgery Kit: Schein Veterinary Catalog, 100–8965.
Jaw prop, large and small: Hauptner, 3360 and 3361.
Large extraction forceps: Martin, 79A; Hauptner, 31510.
Root forceps: Martin, 51; Hauptner, 31531.
Forceps with self-adapting jaws: used as a universal upper and lower forceps: Schein Veterinary Catalog, 100–2405; Martin, 40–534–00.
Root elevator (Bein's elevator): straight, left-curved and right-curved.
Straight: Martin, 559/3; W. Roder, 3208/3; Aesculap, DL 33.
Left-curved: Martin, 561/5.
Right-curved: Martin, 567/4; Hauptner, 32070.
Gouge (straight) about 3 to 5 mm (0.12 to 0.2 in.) wide; Schein Veterinary Catalog, 600–5013; Martin, 1906; Aesculap, CE 230.
Mallet: Schein Veterinary Catalog, 100–6094; Martin, 1241; Aesculap, CE 161.

All forceps with sharp edges or ones that come to a point at the midline of the jaws are not recommended because they will fracture the teeth of small animals, which have weak enamel.

Conservative Treatment

Cotton and dressing pliers: Schein Veterinary Catalog, 100–5709; W. Röder, 1498; Hauptner, 32085 (Fig. 3–1).

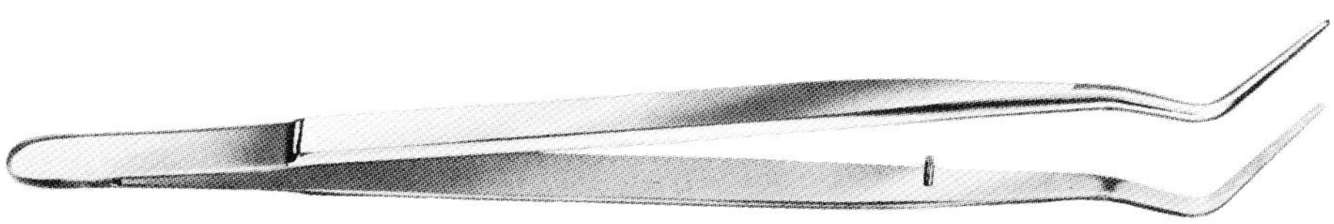

Fig. 3–1. Cotton and dressing pliers.

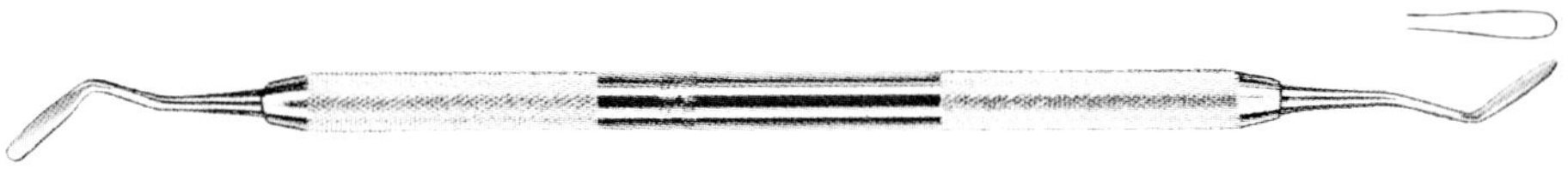

Fig. 3–2. Heidemann spatula.

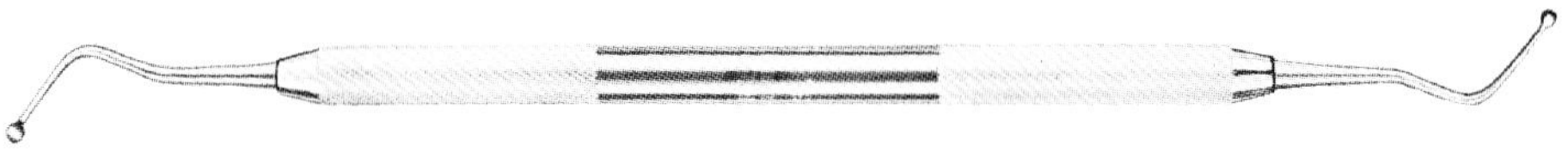

Fig. 3–3. Excavator.

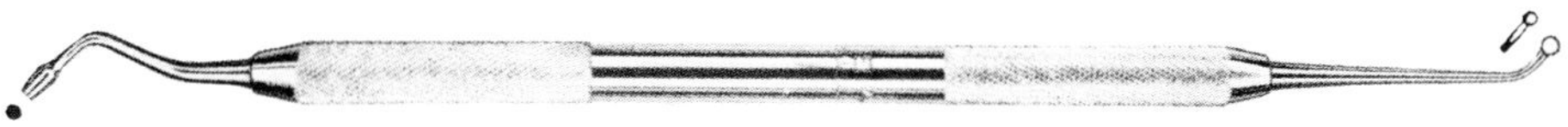

Fig. 3–4. Plugger and burnisher.

Plastic filling instrument: Schein Veterinary Catalog, 100–8645; W. Röder, 1120/2 (Fig. 3–2).

Square broaches and handle 29 mm: Micro-Mega, 4/30.

Excavator: Schein Veterinary Catalog, 100–4065; Maillefer, DE 47/48 (Fig. 3–3).

Pluggers and burnishers: Schein Veterinary Catalog, 100–8754; W. Röder, 1000/23 (Fig. 3–4).

Cold air syringes: Schein Veterinary Catalog, 100–9788.

Amalgam mortar with pestle (in case there is no amalgamator): Schein Veterinary Catalog, 100–0133; Becht, 693.

Medicament bottles: Blue 100–5541, Amber 100–4666, Clear 100–1464, Schein Veterinary Catalog; Kettenbach.

Cotton pellets: Schein Veterinary Catalog, 754–7166, 754–9069, 754–8408; Rauscher, No. 1.

Cotton globules: Hartmann, No. 2.

Glass slab, 10 × 7 mm (0.4 × 0.28 in.): Schein Veterinary Catalog, 100–4432; Kettenbach.

Small cleaning brush for burs: Schein Veterinary Catalog, 365–1135; Komet, 9785.

Instrument trays: Schein Veterinary Catalog, Set A, 100–7436; Set B, 100–8017; Set C, 100–8058.

Periodontal Treatment

Chisel-like scaler: Schein Veterinary Catalog, 100–6703; Aesculap, CE 303; Martin, 1000/60 (Fig. 3–5).

Hooked scaler: Schein Veterinary Catalog, 100–7876; Martin, 10000/72; Aesculap, DB 329 (Fig. 3–6).

Scaling instruments are recommended even if ultrasonic cleaner is at hand!

Scalpel, blades and handle: Schein Veterinary Catalog, 100–7520 and 100–1259.

Gingivectomy instruments: Schein Veterinary Catalog, 100–6840; Martin, 870/1–5 (Fig. 3–7).

For rotating instruments for smoothing and polishing tooth necks and roots, see the next major section of this chapter.

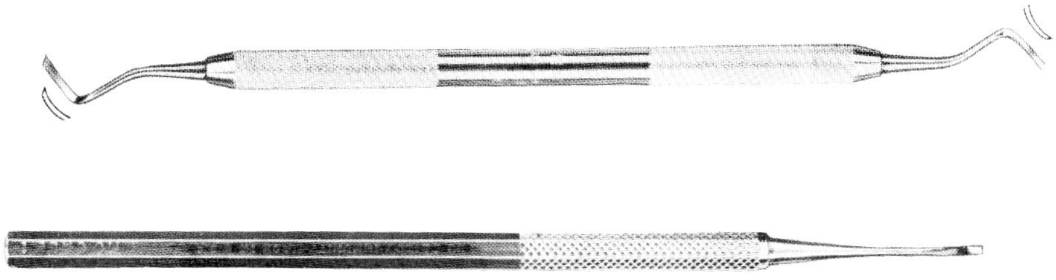

Fig. 3–5. Chisel-like scalers.

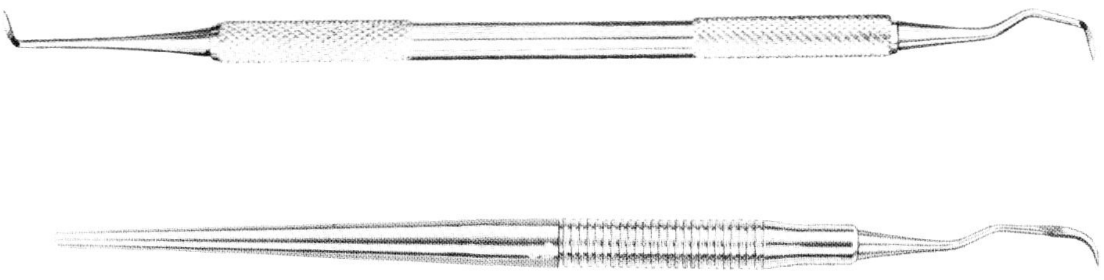

Fig. 3–6. Hooked scalers.

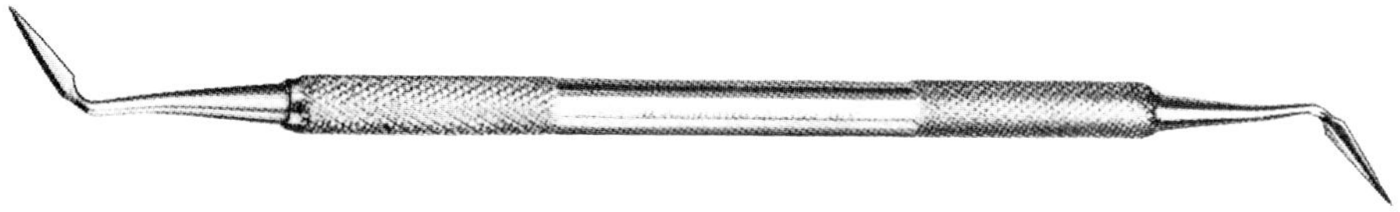

Fig. 3–7. Gingivectomy knife.

Horses and Cattle

Head lamp: Schein Veterinary Catalog, 392–5342.
Mouth lattice: Schein Veterinary Catalog, 100–8702; Hauptner, 3190.
Mouth wedge: Schein Veterinary Catalog, 100–8605; Hauptner, 3690.
Cheek retractor
Tooth rasp: Schein Veterinary Catalog, 100–9056; Hauptner, 32190.
Extraction forceps (special construction; essential: elastic, long handles; wide, flat, concave jaws): Hauptner, 31740.
Chisel, trepanning set
Tooth grinding machine, after Becker, Schouppee (special design).
Instruments for root resection: trepanning set, rotary instruments and drilling engines, as used in small animals.

Rodents

Jaw prop, strong model: Eickemeyer.
Cheek retractor: spatula, Eickemeyer.
Luer rongeur forceps: Schein Veterinary Catalog, 100–7453; Martin, 1830/2; Aesculap, CF 407.

Rotary instruments and drilling engines as used in small animals.

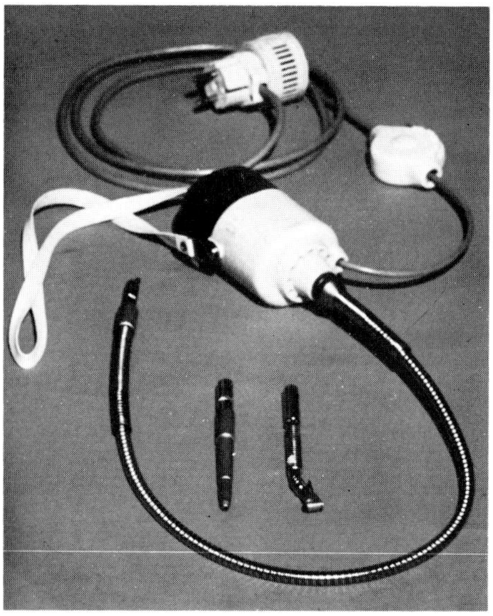

Fig. 3–8. Basic outfit: technician's engine with flexible cable, handpiece, and angle handpiece.

DRILLING ENGINES, BURS AND APPLIANCES

Drilling Engines

Basic Outfit

Technician's engine with pedal starter and flexible cable. (Figs. 3–8, 3–9): Complete Dental Care Unit—VC-30 Schein Veterinary Catalog 100–2787, dental plant Bürmoos U–67–7 together with 5030 and 6700

Contra-angle handpiece: Schein Veterinary Catalog 100–8643, dental plant Bürmoos 704

Advanced Outfit

Giromatic-contra-angle handpiece (for low-speed use of automatic Giro-root canal files in to-and-fro motion): Schein Veterinary Catalog, 100–8931; various firms, Micro-Mega, KaVo, dental plant Bürmoos.

Dental turbine (Fig. 3–10, left)

Advantage: high speed (up to 400,000 r.p.m.), cooling by means of water-spray systems, fast and easy operation.

Disadvantage: cross-contamination by spray-mist, potential subsequent impairment of hearing by whistle signals possible.

Modern combined outfits consist of an air compressor, a turbine, a micromotor, and possibly ultrasonic equipment or an electrotome. In spite of its high initial cost, the outfit is economical when used regularly because of its versatility. A well-tried combined outfit in the line of veterinary dentistry is Esticart (Fig. 3–10, right) (Kaltenbach and Voigt), or the Schein turbine (call for information).

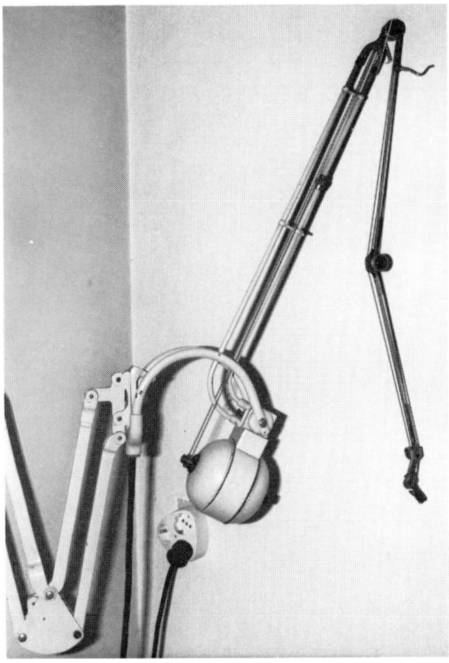

Fig. 3–9. Drilling engine.

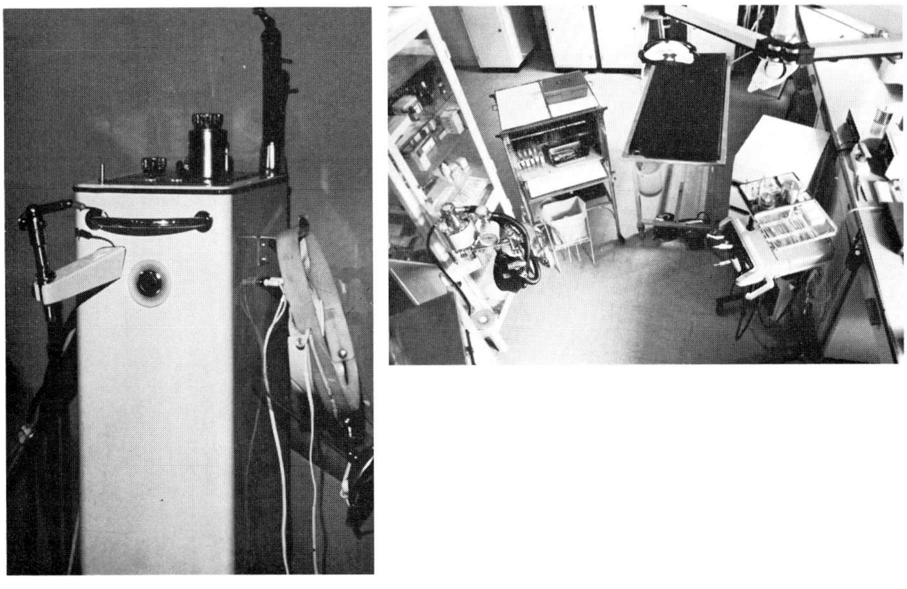

Fig. 3–10. *Left*, Dental turbine. *Right*, Dental Clinic of the Veterinary Medicine Department for Surgery and Ophthalmology, University of Vienna. From left to right: anesthesia apparatus, medicine cabinet, instrument cabinet, treatment bench with flow-off channel, dental surgery light, x-ray apparatus, and complete dental equipment with turbine, micromotor, ultrasonic scaler, hand syringe with six functions; above these are trays for burs and manual instruments.

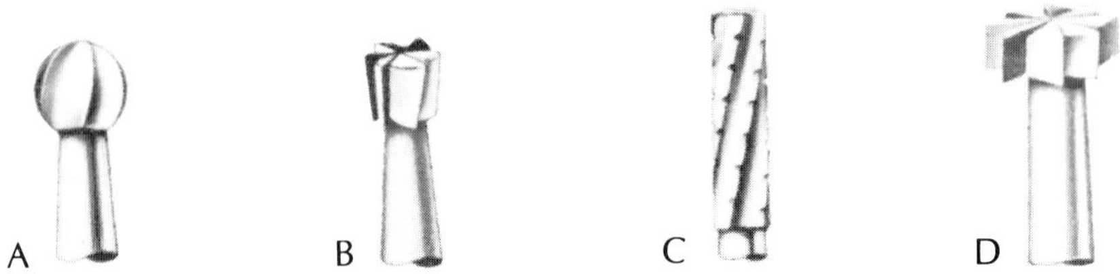

Fig. 3–11. *A*, Rose-head bur; *B*, inverted cone bur; *C*, cross-cut fissure bur; *D*, wheel bur.

Burs, Root Canal Instruments, Finishing and Polishing Instruments

Basic Outfit

Numbers in parentheses refer to ISO code numbers, which have been in international use since 1980.

Contra-angle burs

Rose-head bur, carbide (001001). (Fig. 3–11A): ISO No. 008, US No. 1; Schein Veterinary Catalog, 100–1069; Meisinger; Komet.

Rose-head bur, carbide (001001): ISO No. 012, US No. 4; Schein Veterinary Catalog, 100–1466; Meisinger; Komet.

Rose-head bur, carbide (001001): ISO No. 021, US No. 6; Schein Veterinary Catalog, 100–2351; Meisinger; Komet.

Inverted cone bur, carbide (010001) (Fig. 3–11*B*): ISO No. 008, US No. 34; Schein Veterinary Catalog, 100–7787; Meisinger; Komet.

Inverted cone bur, carbide (010001): ISO No. 012, US No. 35; Schein Veterinary Catalog, 100–1642; Meisinger; Komet.

Inverted cone bur, carbide (010001): ISO No. 021, US No. 37; Schein Veterinary Catalog, 100–8046; US No. 39; Meisinger; Komet.

Cross-cut fissure bur, carbide (107002) (Fig. 3–11C): ISO No. 008, US No. 557; Schein Veterinary Catalog 100–1700; US No. 556; Meisinger; Komet.

Cross-cut fissure bur, carbide (107002): ISO No. 012, US No. 558; Schein Veterinary Catalog, 100–2379; Meisinger, Komet.

Cross-cut fissure bur, carbide (107002): ISO No. 021; Meisinger; Komet.

Wheel bur (040001) (Fig. 3–11*D*): ISO No. 012, US No. 14; Schein Veterinary Catalog, 100–7081; Meisinger; Komet.

Wheel bur (040001): ISO No. 023; Schein Veterinary Catalog, 100–8274; Meisinger; Komet.

Abrasivc head mounted, green (014) (Fig. 3–12*A*): Schein Veterinary Catalog, 195–0087; Meisinger; Komet, shape 613.

Abrasive head mounted, green (041) (Fig. 3–12*B*): Schein Veterinary Catalog, 195–0476; Komet, shape 702; Meisinger, shape 627.

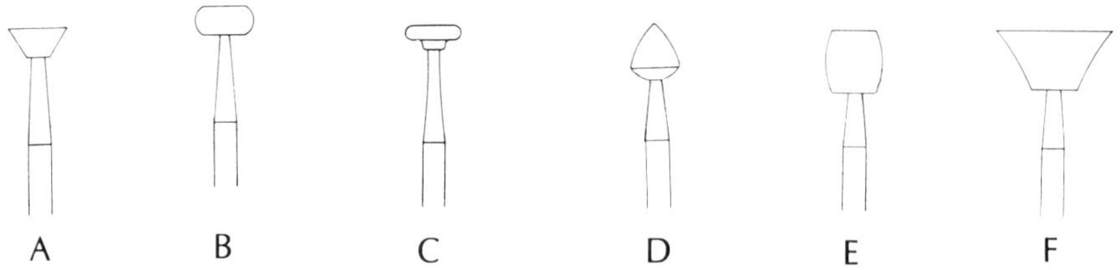

Fig. 3–12. *A* to *F*, Abrasives.

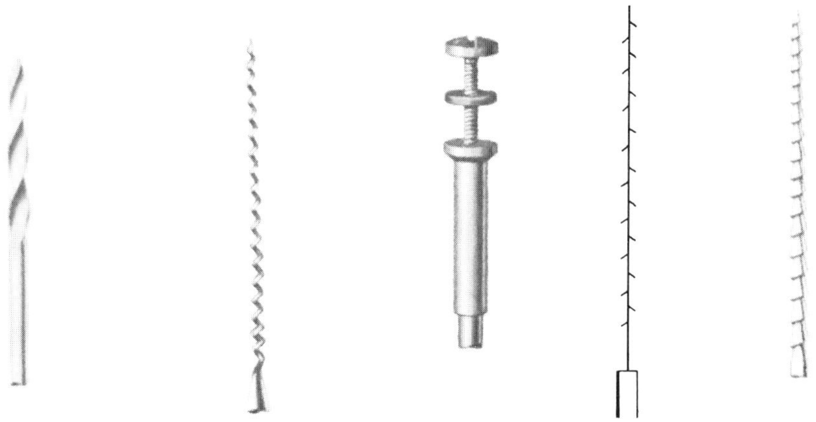

Fig. 3–13. *A*, Root-canal reamer; *B*, root-canal filler; *C*, mandrel for separating disks or abrasive disks; *D*, nerve broach; *E*, root-canal file (Hedstrom file).

Abrasive head mounted, green (042) (Fig. 3–12*C*): Schein Veterinary Catalog, 195–0534; Komet, shape 623; Meisinger, shape 628.

Abrasive head mounted, green (254) (Fig. 3–12*D*): Schein Veterinary Catalog, 195–0718; Komet, shape 658; Meisinger, shape 657.

Abrasive head mounted, green (280) (Fig. 3–12*E*): Schein Veterinary Catalog, 195–0776; Komet, shape 682; Meisinger.

Abrasive head mounted, green (024) (Fig. 3–12*F*): Schein Veterinary Catalog, 195–1136; Komet, shape 727; Meisinger.

Peeso reamers (635459) (Fig. 3–13*A*): Schein Veterinary Catalog, 100–9385; Komet, ISO No. 030, 055, 100; Meisinger, ISO No. 030, 055, 100.

Diamond instruments (160504): Schein Veterinary Catalog, 100–8893 or 100–9228; Komet, shape 8858; Meisinger, 249424, shape 862, ISO No. 016.

Root canal filler (672458) 25 mm (1 in.), (Fig. 3–13*B*): Schein Veterinary Catalog, 100–3791, 928–0883; Meisinger, ISO No. 025, 035, 040; 29 mm (1.16 in.) Komet, ISO No. 025, 035, 040.

Mandrels (603391) (Fig. 3–13C): Schein Veterinary Catalog, 100–0022; Komet; Meisinger.

Barbed broaches, long, assorted, (657455) (Fig. 3–13*D*): Schein Veterinary Catalog, 100–6929, 100–6659, 100–3917, 100–7927; Komet.

Hedstrøm files (653453), 25 and 55 mm (1.00 in. × 2.2 in.) (Fig. 3–13*E*): Schein Veterinary Catalog, 100–0069, 100–4596, 100–5225, 100–2661; Komet, ISO No. 015, 030, 040, 070, 100, 140; (653453) 29 mm (1.16 in.), Meisinger, ISO No. 015, 030, 040.

Paper points for drying the root canal, assorted: Schein Veterinary Catalog, 100–0672, 100–9339; Komet.

Separating disks (Nichrome) for cutting teeth (Fig. 3–14): Schein Veterinary Catalog, 167–2251; Krupp; similar disks manufactured by various firms.

Diamond disks (355504): Schein Veterinary Catalog, 100–2697, 100–6932, 100–0853; Meisinger, ISO No. 220.

Bur stand (Fig. 3–15): Schein Veterinary Catalog, 317–8525; Meisinger, 2011; Komet, 28.

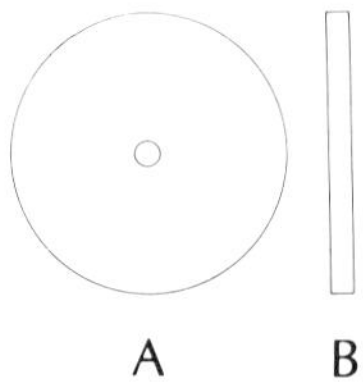

Fig. 3–14. *A* and *B*, Separating disk.

Greenies-brownies: Schein Veterinary Catalog, 195–2822; Hager & Werken; similarly mounted rubber polishing disks, various manufacturers.

Advanced Outfit

Extra long canal files and nerve broaches: Schein Veterinary Catalog, 100–5225, 100–2661; Maillefer, Switzerland: special design on request.

All Burs in FG-Type

Bullet-shaped diamond (Fig. 3–16*A*): Schein Veterinary Catalog, 100–3922, 100–4803; Komet, 249524, ISO No. 021; Meisinger, 250524, ISO No. 018.
Flame-type diamond (Fig. 3–16*B*): Schein Veterinary Catalog, 100–0810; Dica-diamond, 866.
Wheel-shaped bur: Schein Veterinary Catalog, 999–6151; Komet, (040524), ISO No. 023; Meisinger, (068524), ISO No. 031.
Pear-shaped carbide burs (Fig. 3–17*A*): Schein Veterinary Catalog, 100–2817, 100–0928; Komet, (237001), ISO No. 014; Meisinger, (238006), ISO No. 014, US No. 333L.
Fissure bur (107006) (Fig. 3–17*B*): Schein Veterinary Catalog 100–0844; Meisinger, ISO No. 008, US No. 56; Komet.

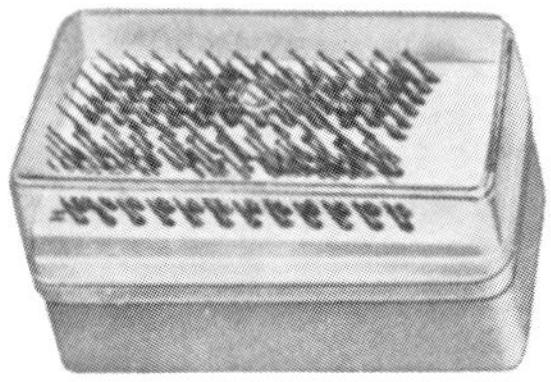

Fig. 3–15. Bur stand.

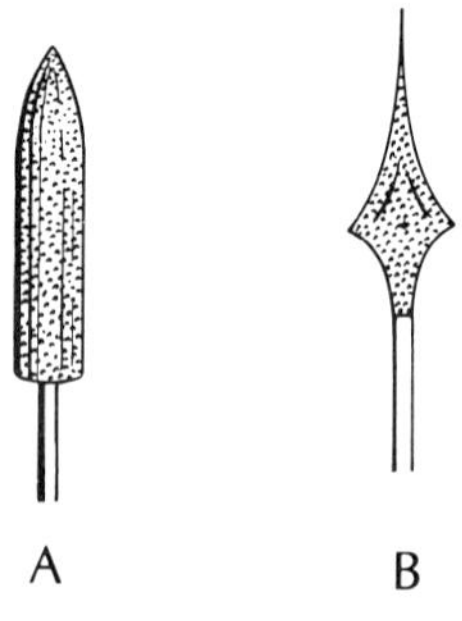

Fig. 3–16. *A*, Bullet-shaped diamond; *B*, flame-type diamond.

Fig. 3–17. *A*, Pear-shaped carbide bur; *B*, fissure bur.

Fissure bur (107006): Schein Veterinary Catalog, 100–6267; Komet, ISO No. 012, US No. 58; Meisinger.
Fissure bur (107006): Meisinger, ISO No. 018, US No. 61; Komet.

Additional Equipment for Low-Speed Drilling Engine, Contra-Angle

Bone cutter (409297) (Fig. 3–18*A*): Schein Veterinary Catalog, 100–3622; Komet, ISO No. 021; Meisinger.
Mandrel (615421) (Fig. 3–18*B*): Schein Veterinary Catalog, 777–3622; Meisinger; Komet.
Composite-disks: Schein Veterinary Catalog, 777–3240, 777–2950, 777–2660. Suited for polishing and smoothing of rough tooth necks and root surfaces. May also be used for polishing of composite material.
TMS-pins (minim and regular) (Fig. 3–19): Schein Veterinary Catalog, 888–5760 (minim), 888–9793 (regular) (TMS = Thread Mate System).

Miscellaneous Dental Equipment

Amalgamator for quick and safe mixing of encapsulated filling materials (not necessary for basic outfit), such as Schein HS1 (Fig. 3–20*A*), Schein Veterinary Catalog, 100–2532.
Ultrasonic equipment for removing tartar (scaling) (Fig. 3–20*B*): Schein Veterinary Catalog, 100–7315 and 167–2142; Sonadent (Bandelin); Cavitron (De Trey); Meditronix (Mediadent); Solid State 100 E (Solid State Systems); Veterinary Ultrasonic Scaler—Schein.
Electrosurgery unit (Fig. 3–21)
Advantage: good view, almost no bleeding.

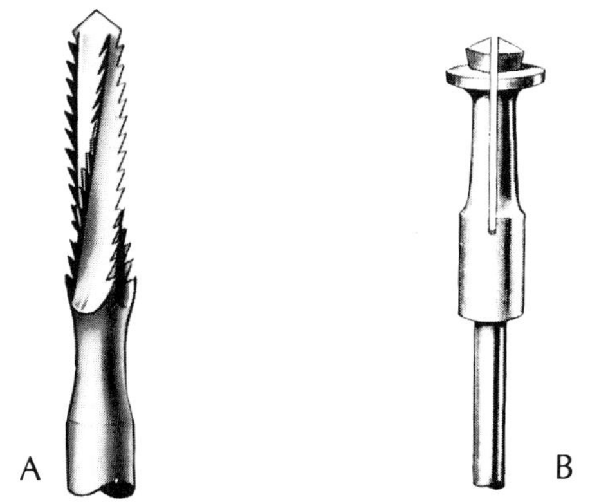

Fig. 3–18. *A*, Bone cutter; *B*, mandrel for composite disks.

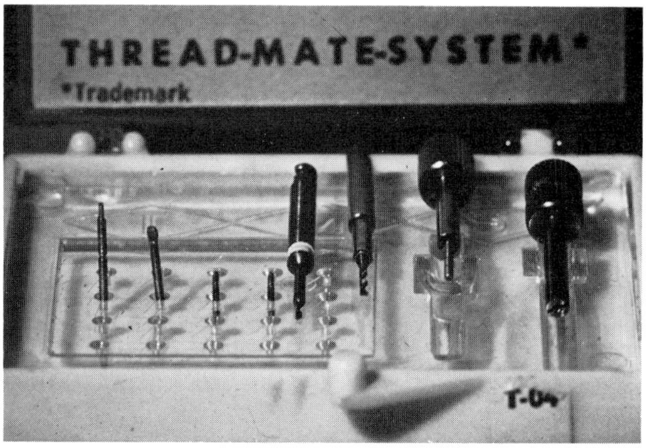

Fig. 3–19. Thread-Mate-System.

Disadvantage: unpleasant odor may develop; improper handling may lead to bone destruction. Particularly suitable for gingivectomy and gingivoplasty. Schein Veterinary Catalog, 295–0874; Martin, 70 D-SE.

MEDICAMENTS AND FILLING MATERIALS

Disinfection of Gingiva and Tooth Surface

Merfen, alcohol 70%, hexachlorophenol preparations, iodine preparations.

Cleaning and Filling the Root Canal

Cleaning

Hypochlorite for cleaning the root canal chemically and 3% H_2O_2 for subsequent neutralization of hypochlorite: Schein Veterinary Catalog, 100–7562 and 472–3516.

Camphorated chlorphenol solution: Schein Veterinary Catalog, 100–3677.

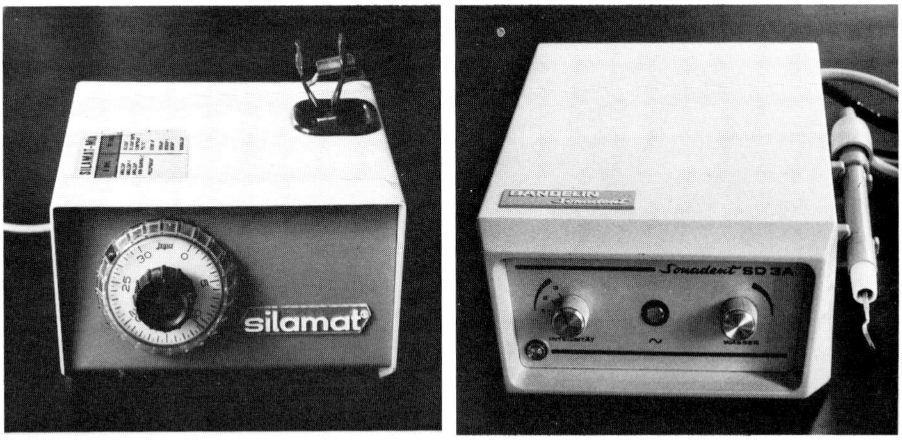

Fig. 3–20. *A*, Amalgamator; *B*, ultrasonic unit.

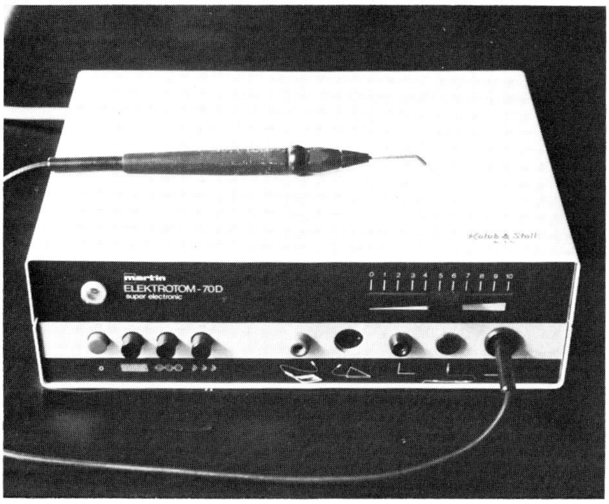

Fig. 3–21. Electrosurgery unit.

Filling

N_2 (for gangrenous pulps): Schein Veterinary Catalog, 117–8362; De Trey, AH 26; Espe, Diaket.

Gutta-percha points for all root canal filling materials: Schein Dental Catalog, 100–9997 and 100–1871.

Mortal Amputation

Dr. Gonser mummification globules are well-suited for filling the pulp canals in horses after apicoectomy.

Direct (Vital Amputation) or Indirect Capping of Vital Pulp

Calxyl-paste red: calcium hydroxide (pasty consistency), Oco.

Ledermix: a mixture of cortisone and antibiotics as paste or cement, Lederle.

Reocap E. (provided a mixer for capsules is available): calcium hydroxide in fast-hardening cement, Vivadent.

Hydroxiline: for indirect capping, Schein Veterinary Catalog, 514–9199.

Zinc Oxide-Eugenol: Schein Veterinary Catalog, 100–7743 and 100–3688.

Hemostatic: solution of epinephrine and hydrogen peroxide 3%.

Dycal (Caulk), Schein Veterinary Catalog, 222–3482.

Pulp Protection Materials

Intermediate layers are needed to protect pasty pulp-capping agents (vital amputation) or root-canal fillings from pressure during plugging and condensing. These materials are recommended also with composite fillings.

Zinc phosphate cements: Schein Veterinary Catalog, 100–1492 and 100–6200; Vivadent, Tenet-cement, powder No. 7 and fluid; Richter & Hoffmann, Harvard Cement; Vivadent, Reocap.

Filling Materials

The thermal coefficient of expansion and the abrasive characteristics of filling materials should be similar to those of the tooth tissue. Also desirable are low water absorption, impermeability to bacteria, and resistance to corrosion. If thermal conductivity is high, as with amalgam, or if a chemical tissue incompatibility exists, as with residual monomers of composite materials, an insulating relining will be necessary to protect the living pulp.

Amalgams

Silver amalgam is commonly employed, whereas copper amalgam alloys are rarely used.

Silver amalgam alloys are available at various firms: Schein Veterinary Catalog, 100–0037 and 100–7863 (mercury). Chips of a silver-tin alloy containing 50 to 70% silver are alloyed by grinding with mercury in a mortar: this alloy is particularly recommendable if cavities cannot be kept dry, as in caries in cats. This alloy is also available in convenient capsules, premeasured for use in amalgamators; an example is Amalcap (Vivadent).

In **non-gamma-2 amalgam,** the corroding phase, or the so-called gamma-2 phase, has been eliminated; the filling therefore possesses greater durability. It is a first-class filling material for dry cavities. Moisture such as in the form of blood, leads to expansion of the amalgam and destruction of the filling. Non-gamma-2 amalgam is less suited for bleeding carious cavities in cats. In dogs, the following have proved useful: Dispersalloy (Johnson & Johnson) and Amalcap non-gamma-2 (Vivadent). Both are available in capsules premeasured for use in amalgamators. Manual blending of activated capsules in a mortar is recommended with non-gamma-2 amalgam only, particularly Dispersalloy. Schein Veterinary Catalog, 100–2362 (amalgam) and 100–7863 (mercury).

Plastic Materials

Compared to amalgam, these materials possess low thermal conductivity, although the border seal does not always reach the density of amalgam because of polymerization contraction. Acrylates are less suitable because of their high thermal coefficient of expansion.

Epoxy-resin derivatives of the bis-GMA type are recommended. Composite materials contain inorganic filling materials to increase abrasion strength and to decrease the coefficient of expansion. The smaller the filling compound, the easier it is to polish and the more resistant it is to abrasion (boron silicates, quartz crystals, glass fibers).

Autopolymerizing composites: Schein Veterinary Catalog, 100–1673; Johnson & Johnson, Adaptic; Kulzer, Estic; Vivadent, Isopast; Lee Pharmaceuticals, Epoxydent.

Ultraviolet or visible light composites (needed for special techniques): Schein Veterinary Catalog, 555–6102; De Trey, Nuva system; Johnson & Johnson, Fotofil; Kulzer, Estilux and Durafill.

PREPARATION OF THE TOOTH

Materials that cannot be glued onto the enamel must be anchored in a mechanical way as a filling in the tooth itself, by one of the three following methods: (1) ensuring that the inner dimension of the cavity is larger than the outer dimension (Fig. 3–22*A*); (2) anchorage by means of TMS pins (Fig. 3–22*B*); or (3) Dovetail preparation (Fig. 3–22C).

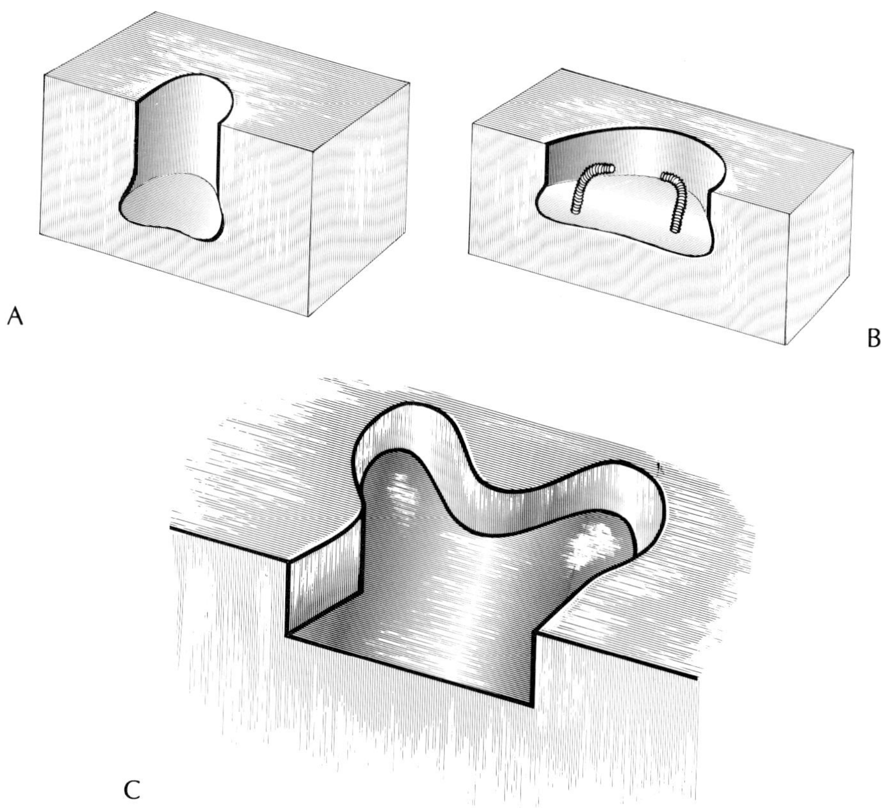

Fig. 3–22. *A*, Inverted conical cavity preparation for anchoring fillings; *B*, anchorage by means of Thread-Mate-System pins; *C*, dovetail preparation.

Principles of Cavity Preparation

First, the tooth surface should be cleaned of calculus and plaque and disinfected. Insertion of the bur into the angle handpiece and the correct operating position are demonstrated in Figure 3–23. Cutting of the carious tooth with a rose-head bur is shown in Figure 3–24. Because of heat production, one should not drill on one point for too long, but rather use gentle pressure in a curving or circular motion. Drilling should be performed in a waltzlike rhythm: drill for one beat, pause for two beats. It is essential to have a clear view of the bottom of the cavity to be drilled.

Inverted conical burs should be used to enlarge the cavity to the conical shape desired (Fig. 3–25*A*). The cavity's diameter should be larger than 3 mm (0.12 in.). The sharp edges inside should be rounded off (Fig. 3–25*B*).

Carious teeth should be drilled with a fissure bur, to ensure that no retention sites for food are left and thus to diminish the danger of secondary caries (Fig. 3–26).

Preparing for Root Treatment

One should round off the edges of the root-canal entrance with a rose-head bur or a diamond barrel. The spoon excavator is used to determine whether any

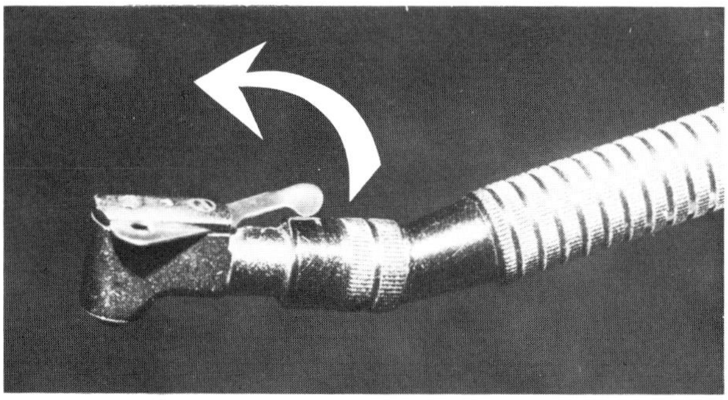
A

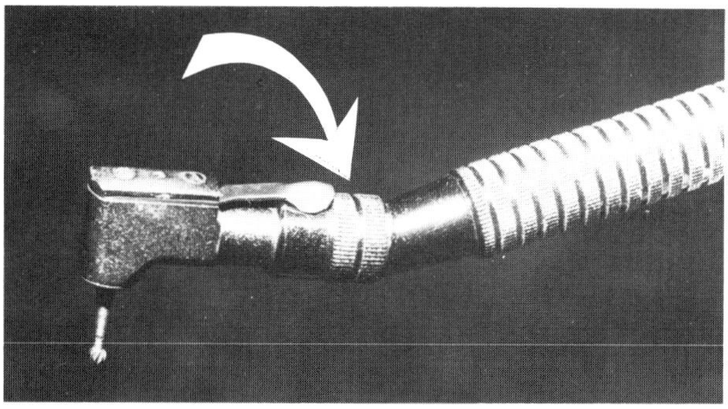
B

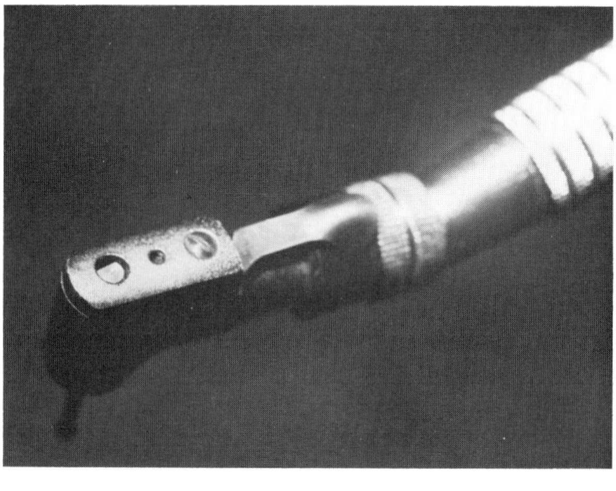
C

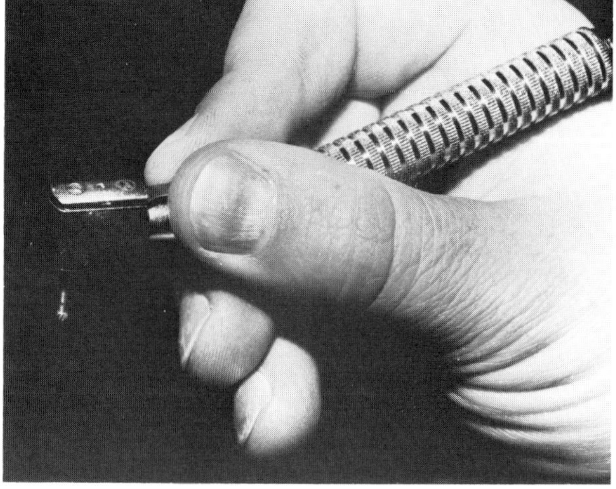
D

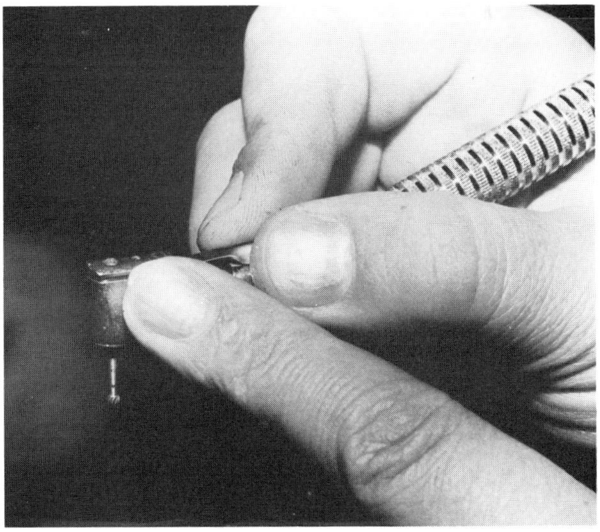

E

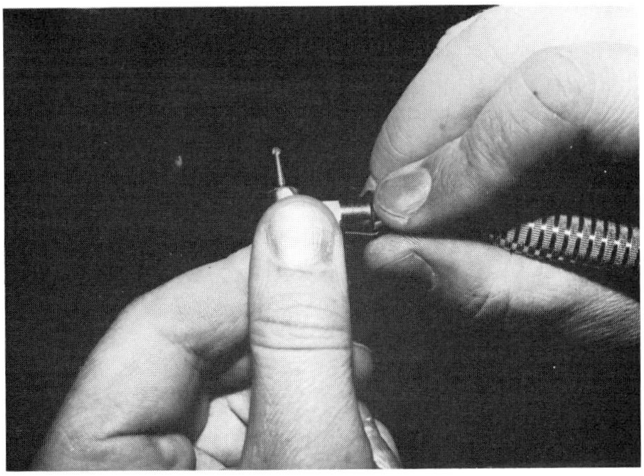

F

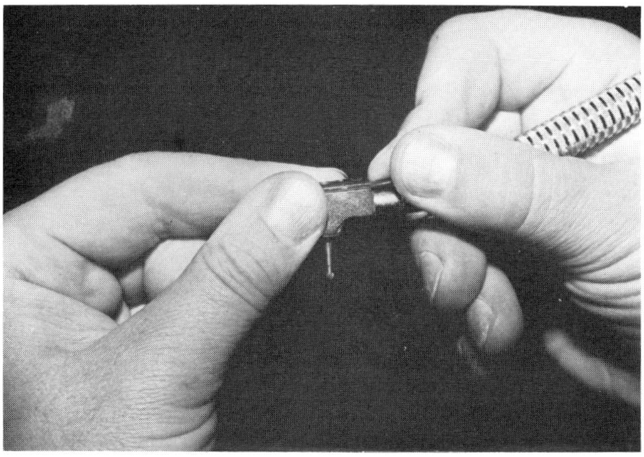

G

Fig. 3–23. *A,* Before inserting the bur, the bolting lever (arrow) on the angle handpiece must be turned sideways. *B,* The lever (arrow) is set straight for bolting the bur. *C,* After correct bolting, the bur base is visible in the hole of the angle handpiece. *D,* The angle handpiece held correctly. *E,* To ensure precise drilling, the bur head may be supported by the forefinger. *F,* One should use both hands for drilling upward. *G,* One should use both hands for an especially precise preparation.

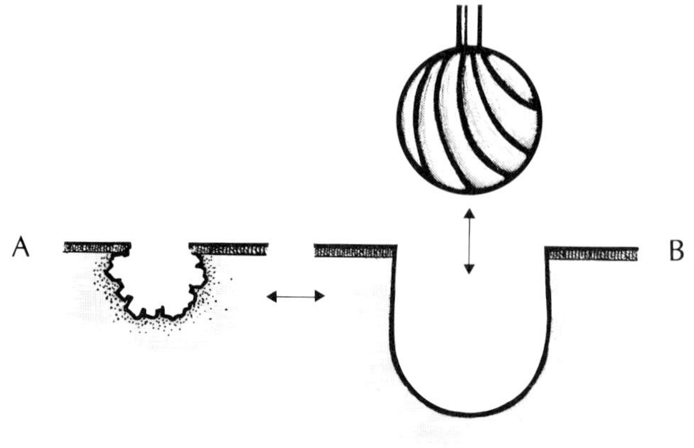

Fig. 3–24. *A*, Caries; *B*, tooth after removal of caries with a rose-head bur.

carious dentin remains to be removed and whether shoulders or bacterial-retention sites are present.

The cavity should be cleansed with a disinfectant solution or with 70% ethanol before one inserts the filling. The cavity should be dried with an air-blower syringe.

If one cannot adequately anchor the filling by preparing an inverted conical cavity or by inserting TMS pins, horizontal filling retainers can be drilled in dovetail fashion.

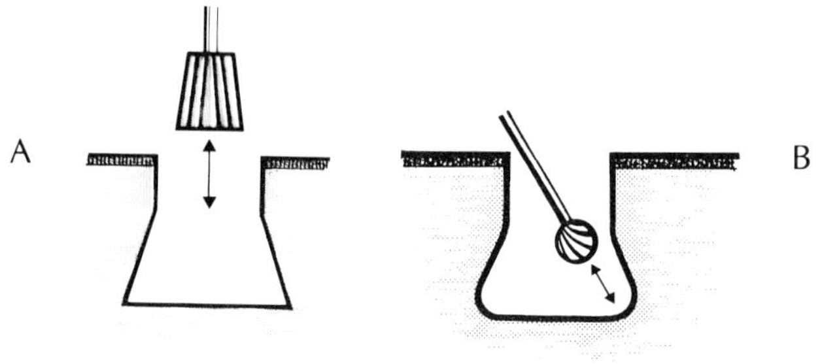

Fig. 3–25. *A*, Cavity enlarged with a conical bur; *B*, rounding of sharp edges.

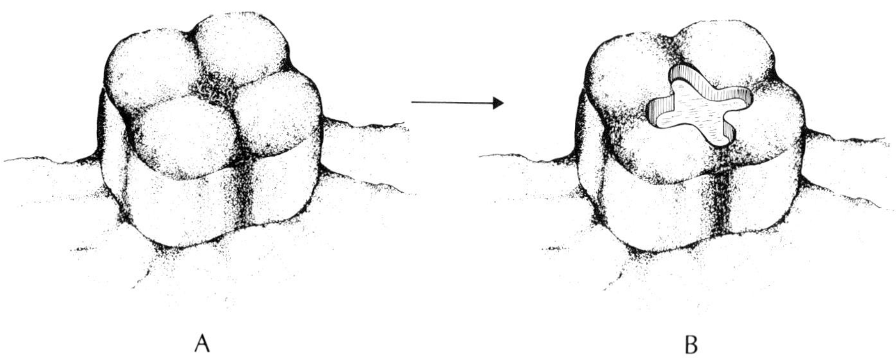

Fig. 3–26. *A*, Carious tooth; *B*, tooth drilled with a fissure bur.

FILLING OF THE TOOTH

Amalgam

Amalgam should only be used to fill cavities, not to build up crowns.

Mixing

Mercury should be added to the silver-tin chips drop by drop, while one is constantly grinding, until a homogeneous compound that is not too soft is formed. Then the amalgam should be rolled between the fingertips under strong pressure, to form a small ball and to squeeze out any surplus mercury. One should continue to knead the amalgam until a crunching sound is heard, similar to the sound of making a snowball. When in doubt, amalgam should be damp because it is easier to model; dry amalgam crumbles.

Caution: Mercury vapor is poisonous, so one must not drop any mercury.

Mechanical Mixing. When the encapsulated amalgam has been activated, by pressing or by pulling the capsule knob according to the manufacturer's instructions, one should put the capsules into the amalgamator. In 5 to 10 seconds, the amalgam is ready for use.

When using non-gamma-2 amalgam, one should not touch the material (because of perspiration), but rather administer it with an amalgam gun.

Application

A small portion of amalgam is squeezed onto the amalgam carrier and is inserted into the cavity layer by layer. One should condense each layer (about 1 to 3 mm or 0.04 to 0.12 in. thick) under pressure with the condenser, squeezing out surplus mercury. Condensing should be done carefully toward the cavity flange because strength, border seal, and durability depend on it.

The surface of the filling is then modeled and smoothed by a spatula. Occlusion should then be checked and remodeled if necessary. Hardening occurs within 2 hours, but final hardening takes a month or so.

Polishing

One should polish the filling with a polishing rubber cup in a few days, or the owner can do it with a pencil eraser. Plaque formation is delayed by the smooth surface, and durability is secured.

Composite Resin

These materials may be used as filling compounds and in restoration with the enamel-etch technique.

Mixing

Composites are mixed from two pastes with a plastic spatula and should be applied within a minute. The cavity wall should be clean and dry. Touching the material after application may disturb the polymerization process.

With some filling compounds, such as Adaptic, one can control the viscosity by using different proportions of paste or fluid. These preparations have the advantage of being easy to apply as well as the disadvantage of reduced resistance to abrasion if one uses too much fluid and thereby decreases the amount of inorganic filling material.

Composites should be applied with plastic spatulas only; metallic instruments should not be used because of tarnishing. Opaquer may be used in some preparations to obtain a porcelain-white shade, which is advantageous in young dogs and is preferred by animal owners.

Hardening of the composite material occurs without heating in 3 to 5 minutes. When the material is taken out of a refrigerator, polymerization may be retarded up to 8 minutes. As a remedial measure, one can mix the desired portion on a heated glass slab, which must be cleaned with acetone or chloroform immediately after use.

For storage and durability, one should follow the manufacturer's instructions. Composites may be kept in a refrigerator at a temperature of 4° C for about a year and in a freezer for several years. Isopast has to be kept at room temperature. Hardened composites may be worked up in 15 to 20 minutes, according to the manufacturer's directions, but our own experience suggests that they may be used immediately after hardening. A high-luster polish may be achieved by coating the surface with a glazing varnish. Missing inorganic filling materials reduce the durability of a coating by 6 to 18 months. When finishing the filling or building the crown, occlusion should always be checked and, if necessary, adjusted and corrected.

DENTAL IMPRESSION MODELS (CASTS)

These models are necessary for corrective orthodontia and producing cast (gold) crowns.

Materials

Basic Outfit

Alginate impression: Schein Veterinary Catalog, 100–5292.

These impressions are inexpensive and save time; however, they are inaccurate in many cases and cannot be used in small livestock because of divergingly curved canine teeth. Impressions must be quickly reinforced with plaster, for which an impression tray is desirable.

Alginate should be mixed with water, taken up by an impression tray, and pressed onto the dentition. When hardened, a few minutes later, the impression, which has little elasticity and no great tensile strength, may be removed. It should be promptly reinforced with plaster lest it be deformed when it dries.

Advanced Outfit

Two-phase silicone impression technique for precision impressions (see Fig. 3–27*A*), Schein Veterinary Catalog 123–2959.

First phase: Hard plastic impression compound.

Application. A portion ranging from the size of a plum to the size of an apple should be mixed with the appropriate number of drops of hardener (one must wear gloves), pressed onto the dentition, and modeled. In 3 to 5 minutes, the impression, which is elastic and possesses tensile strength, may be removed. One should clean the remaining impression material from the patient's teeth.

Second phase: precision impression compound.

Application: One should mix according the the manufacturer's instructions; the liquid material should be applied onto the impression that was just removed.

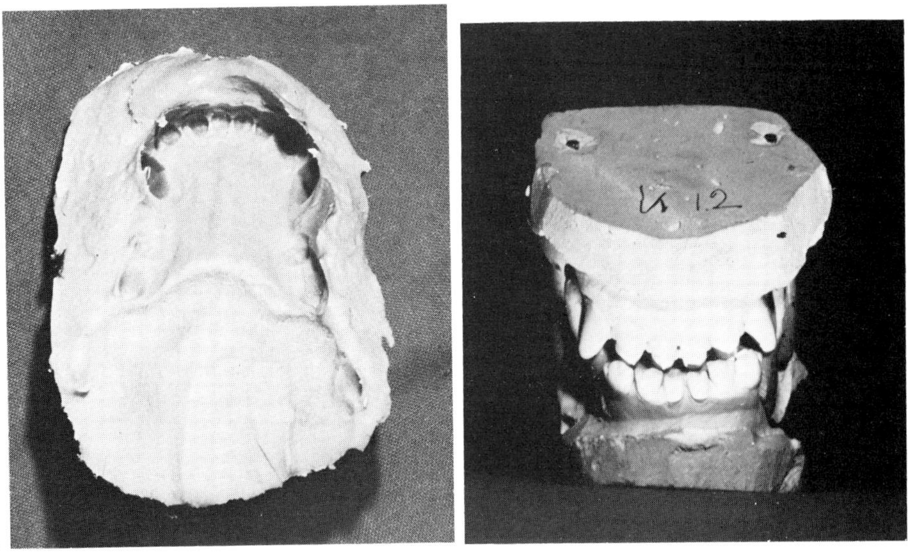

A B

Fig. 3–27. *A*, Silicone impression; *B*, plaster cast of dentition.

The impression should again be firmly pressed onto the patient's dentition. Remove 3 to 5 minutes later. The impression is an exact reproduction of the entire dentition or the individual tooth. The plaster-wash impression may be accomplished 1 to 2 days later.

Plaster Cast

Casting plaster: Dentstone Yellow (Modern Material), Schein Veterinary Catalog 569–8553; Glastone, Ransom & Randolph.

Application. Powder should be added to the water and stirred until the mixture reaches the consistency of whipped cream. As few air bubbles as possible should be allowed to develop. Then the plaster paste should be inserted into the impression, which should be repeatedly knocked against a hard base until all air bubbles have escaped. Deep cavities, such as those formed by the canine teeth, should be checked by poking with an explorer to see if the filling is free of air bubbles. Plaster should be inserted layer by layer until the impression is filled. In 30 to 180 minutes, after the setting heat has decreased, the impression compound should be removed carefully from the plaster cast. The plastic compound should not be pulled off, but rather should be cut away layer by layer with a sharp knife. One must be especially careful not to damage the canine teeth. The plaster cast can be handed over to the dental technician, or it may be used as a working model in one's own workshop (Fig. 3–27*B*). It is advisable for those who are less experienced to make two impressions and two plaster casts. The plaster cast should be coated with an insulating agent so that the appliance worked on it can be removed again.

TECHNOLOGY OF ORTHODONTICS

Materials

Steel wire, spring-hard, 0.8 mm (0.03 in.): Dentaurum No. 522–070, Forestadent No. 213–8080.

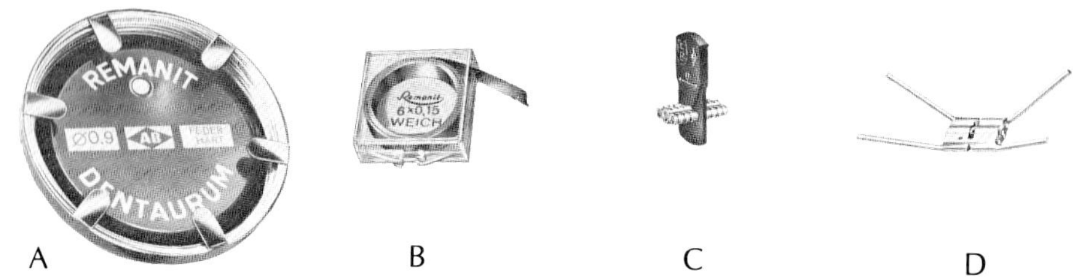

Fig. 3–28. *A* to *D*, orthodontic wire band material and expansion screw devices.

Steel wire, 1.2 mm (0.048 in.): Dentaurum, No. 522–120; Forestadent, No. 213–7120.

Steel wire, 2.0 mm (0.08 in.): Schein Veterinary Catalog 100–2684, 100–2468, 100–3401; Dentaurum, No. 522 (Fig. 3–28*A*).

Band material for banding anchor teeth or bridge abutment teeth: 6.0 mm × 0.15 mm (0.24 in. × 0.006 in.), Dentaurum, No. 804–060 (Fig. 3–28*B*).

Welding apparatus: (Microflame Torch), small welding unit with butane or oxygen cartridges (not available everywhere because of criminal misuse).

Steel gold solder, available at local refineries: Ogussa, DWL 801.

Flux: Ogussa, Oxynon.

Sturdy encased expansion screws: 9 to 11 mm wide (0.36 to 0.44 in.): Dentaurum, 601–114; Forestadent, 121–0922; Forestadent, 131–1111.

Expansion screw 13 mm (0.52 in.) wide: Dentaurum, 601–112; Forestadent, 151–1322.

Expansion screw 15 mm (0.6 in.) wide: Dentaurum 601–110, Forestadent 151–1522 (Fig. 3–28*C*).

Expansion screws often have a self-locking thread so that the screw cannot turn back easily by itself.

Hyrax, expansion screws after Biedermann, 13 to 14 mm (0.52 to 0.64 in.): Dentaurum, 602–810; Forestadent, 167–1422.

Hyrax screws, 20 to 22 mm (0.8 to 0.88 in.): Dentaurum, 602–813; Forestadent, 167–2022 (Fig. 3–28*D*).

Sheldon-pliers: Schein Veterinary Catalog, 100–9340; Dentaurum, 003–007; Forestadent, 501–0206 (Fig. 3–29*A*).

Roundnosed pliers: Schein Veterinary Catalog, 100–3656; Forestadent, 501–0403 (Fig. 3–29*B*).

Aderer pliers: Schein Veterinary Catalog, 100–3153; Dentaurum, 003–200; Forestadent, 501–0701 (Fig. 3–29*C*).

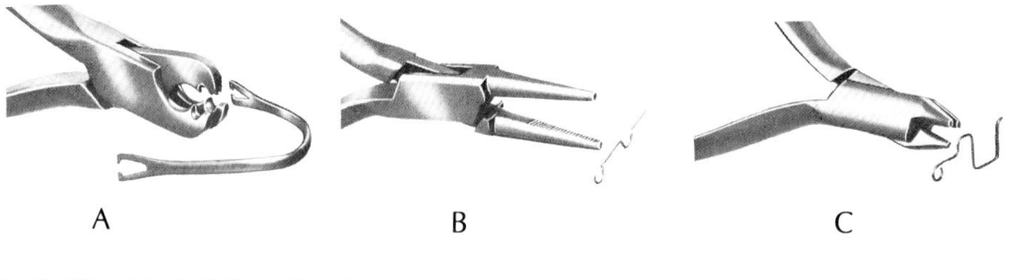

Fig. 3–29. *A* to *C*, Orthodontic pliers.

Plastic cold-curing compound (acrylic), clear: Schein Veterinary Catalog, 125–4890; Dentaurum, 160–012 and 161–000.
Releasing agent: Schein Veterinary Catalog, 123–3028; Dentaurum, 162–800.

Technique

Individual teeth may be moved by spring attachments or screws. Groups of teeth may be moved by means of the compressive or tensile stress of a wire arch with activating loops or by means of expansion screws.

Jaw crowding is relieved by using sturdy encased screws. See Chapter 5 for a discussion of the production of orthodontic appliances.

Soldering

Both metal parts to be soldered should be thoroughly cleaned, coated with a thin layer of flux, and mounted on a holder in the desired position. Light the soldering torch and add oxygen until the soldering flame has reached a temperature of about 2600° C (blue flame with a white core).

Heat both metallic parts until they are red-hot, then hold the steel gold solder in the flame for a short time until a drop of solder is dissolved on both metallic parts. Remove the flame and solder immediately. Allow to cool. Then polish the oxidized metal with a rubber cap or with a brush and abrasive agent.

Insertion of the Mechanism

The metal frame is cemented onto the enamel surface of the bridge abutment teeth using composites with the adhesion technique (see Chap. 6). Removable appliances cannot be used in dogs.

Bibliography: 4, 6, 8, 9, 11, 18, 21, 23, 38, 39, 43, 52

4

Abnormalities in Dentition and Change of Teeth

NORMAL CHANGE AND ERUPTION OF TEETH

In carnivores, the shedding of deciduous teeth and the eruption of permanent teeth occur between the ages of 5 and 7 months and, as a rule, do not cause any general symptoms.

A loosened deciduous premolar may occasionally adhere to the gingiva and may be turned in a transverse position. Wide opening of the mouth cavity, scratching the cheek, sticking out the tongue, salivation, and impaired food intake indicate a disturbance in the mouth cavity. Passive closure of the jaws may be blocked.

The differential diagnosis includes impacted foreign bodies and inflammatory processes within the region of teeth, gingiva, tongue, and pharynx; fracture of the mandible and jaw luxation must also be considered.

In herbivores, the change and eruption of posterior teeth, between the ages of 6 and 54 months, often cause disturbances. Shedding the deciduous premolars leaves a wide, deep, gingival lesion in which food may become impacted. Marginal gingivitis thus develops and may spread to the permanent tooth. In the end, this disorder manifests itself as alveolar periostitis or fistula. Even in a less-drastic course, the temporary inflammatory chewing dysfunction causes food refusal and general discomfort. Partly loosened dental caps occasionally assume a transverse position and may irritate the tongue or cheek.

Treatment

It is easy to remove a loosened deciduous tooth; healing of the gingiva is furthered by antiseptic irrigation or topical application of antiseptic or mildly astringent fluids. One should feed soft food for some time and remove the loosened remnants of teeth.

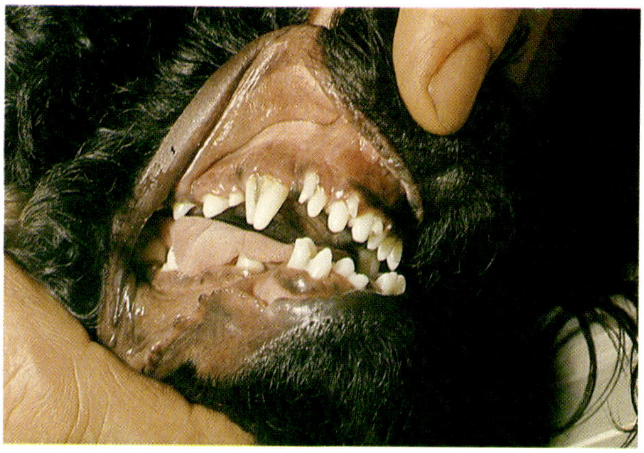

Fig. 4–1. Persistent canines and incisors in a dog.

PERSISTENT DECIDUOUS TEETH

Signs and Symptoms

A smaller, white deciduous tooth often remains next to or in place of a permanent one. One or more persistent deciduous teeth may be present. They are often symmetrically arranged, such as both canine teeth in the maxilla of dogs, as an additional dental arch in the incisor region, or rarely, in the premolar region (Fig. 4–1). Persistent deciduous teeth may give the impression of polyodontia (Fig. 4–2). The x-ray picture shows the deciduous tooth with its shorter, slender root, or the not-yet-erupted permanent tooth can often be seen (see the section on tooth retention).

In any case, it is recommended that the patient's dentition be radiographed if, according to the animal's age, a deciduous tooth should have changed and the permanent tooth has not yet erupted. These "missing" permanent teeth are displaced tooth germs that may hinder the roots of other teeth when they grow or may later form lesions of the jaw in the form of follicular cysts or tumors. Persistent deciduous teeth of herbivores abrade much more strongly than per-

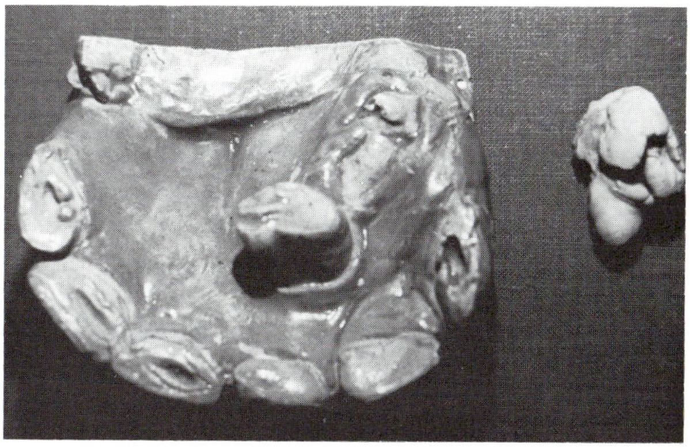

Fig. 4–2. Persistent incisors in the mandible of a horse. The germs of the permanent teeth have been distally displaced by a fracture of the mandible. To the right is the malformed I2.

manent teeth; for example, the mark of a persistent incisor in horses completely disappears, but it is still clearly visible on the adjacent permanent teeth.

Food is frequently impacted between persistent deciduous and permanent teeth. Parodontitis and calculus formation are equally frequent; a retained deciduous tooth occasionally obstructs and displaces a growing permanent tooth.

Cause

A deciduous tooth is persistent when its root is not resorbed under the pressure of the erupting permanent tooth, and the deciduous tooth is not pushed out of its alveolus. This phenomenon occurs when the erupting permanent tooth is not present at all or when it pushes out at the wrong place or in the wrong direction. If the deciduous tooth is not in a normal position, the permanent tooth may slide past it. Persistent deciduous teeth may also be found in older animals.

Dogs of some small breeds, such as Pomeranians, Yorkshire terriers, fox terriers, poodles, and dachshunds, have multiple deciduous tooth persistency of the canines, the incisors, and more rarely, the premolars; a genetic predisposition is assumed. Such displacement of embryonic tooth germs is less common in other animals and is, in most cases, restricted to individual teeth; even casual traumatic injuries may be causative factors. This situation has often been observed in the incisor region in horses as a sequela of obliquely healed jaw fractures. The deciduous tooth is in the right position and is fully efficient, but is shed prematurely.

Treatment

One should extract the persistent deciduous tooth when it is useless, when it hinders the permanent tooth, or when it is the cause of further pathologic symptoms. As a rule, these indications apply to carnivores, in which a slightly displaced permanent tooth can be correctly positioned by orthodontic treatment.

According to its shape and position a permanent tooth may also cause disturbances in chewing. Such a tooth should be carefully extracted, thus ensuring that the persistent deciduous tooth can assume its function for some time. It is often advisable to grind down the displaced teeth, or even to undertake root treatment, to render these teeth useful in chewing.

The persistent deciduous tooth should be extracted as soon as the permanent tooth becomes visible, provided that the corresponding deciduous tooth does not show any signs of being loose or resorbed. Such is the case with small breeds of dogs 5 to 8 months old. If the permanent tooth grows orthognathically, the persistent tooth need not be extracted for a few weeks; meanwhile, the root of the deciduous tooth will be partially resorbed.

Extraction Technique

Persistent deciduous teeth in carnivores are fragile; extraction using forceps usually results in crown or root fractures. It is therefore recommended to loosen the tooth with Bein's elevator, which must be placed carefully between the alveolar wall and the tooth. Equally suitable is the incision of the gingiva above the long root of the persistent canine tooth; this root is labial to the permanent tooth and is almost straight, in contrast to the visible crown. The outer alveolar wall is then removed using a gouge and mallet. The exposed root can then be

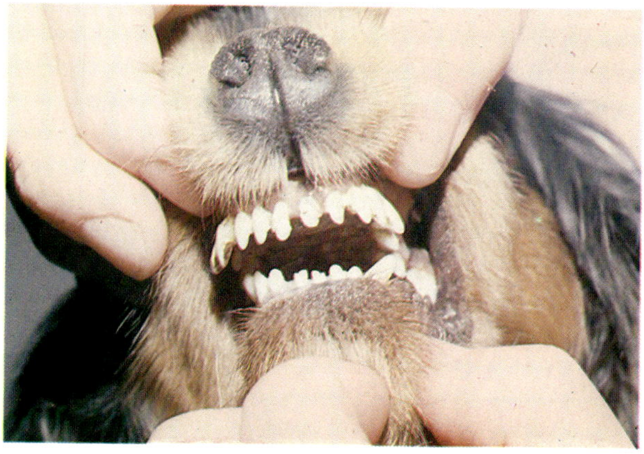

Fig. 4–3. Polyodontia in a 2-year-old dog.

easily loosened from its socket. If, in spite of all these precautions, a root breaks, reasonable efforts must be made to remove the remaining root structure. Although the body usually resorbs retained root fragments, it occasionally treats them as a foreign body, causing considerable inflammation. Substantial damage to the periodontium of the permanent tooth may result.

A roentgenogram can show the condition and position of the root portion, as well as the inflammatory process. Persistent deciduous teeth in herbivores are extracted in the same manner as in carnivores.

POLYODONTIA, SUPERNUMERARY TEETH, AND HYPERDONTIA

Unlike an apparent polyodontia caused by persistent deciduous teeth, we are concerned here with an increased number of equal teeth (Fig. 4–3). Clinically, the differentiation between a persistent deciduous tooth and a permanent tooth is not always clear but it may be facilitated by an x-ray examination that shows the length and the size of the root. The first premolar (wolf tooth), which occasionally erupts in the maxilla of horses, does not meet the criteria for polyodontia because a regular tooth germ is involved in its eruption.

The supernumerary teeth stand next to or in the molar region and may have no counterparts on the opposing side. The posterior teeth of the part of jaw in question appear to be elongated mesially or distally. Thus, in herbivores, lack of abrasion results in abnormal elongation; if exsuperantia dentis develops, then the consequent pressure in the opposing jaw may lead to necrosis (Fig. 4–4).

Food may become impacted between the supernumerary tooth next to the molar region and the regular tooth, and putrefaction and gingivitis may result. Even the movement of the tongue may be hindered, and painful erosions in the buccal mucosa may develop. Supernumerary third tooth germs may be impacted without evidence of polyodontia. Such teeth may have abnormal shapes, or they may grow together with other teeth (twin teeth, Fig. 4–5).

Cause

Division or double disposition of one or several tooth germs is the source of extra teeth. This phenomenon is common in brachygnathous dogs and in the posterior dental region of herbivores.

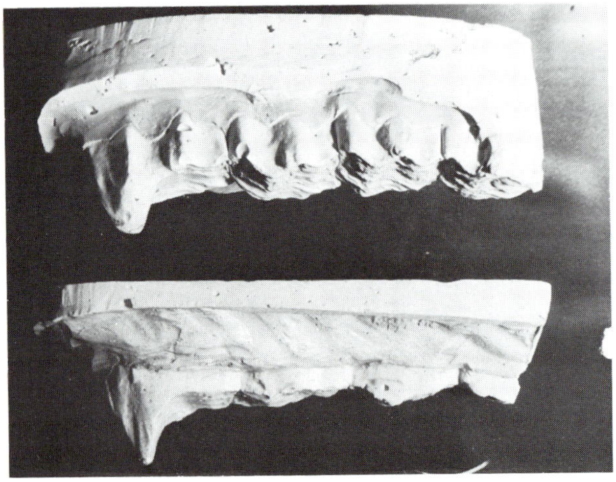

Fig. 4–4. Exsuperantia dentis caused by teeth rows of unequal length.

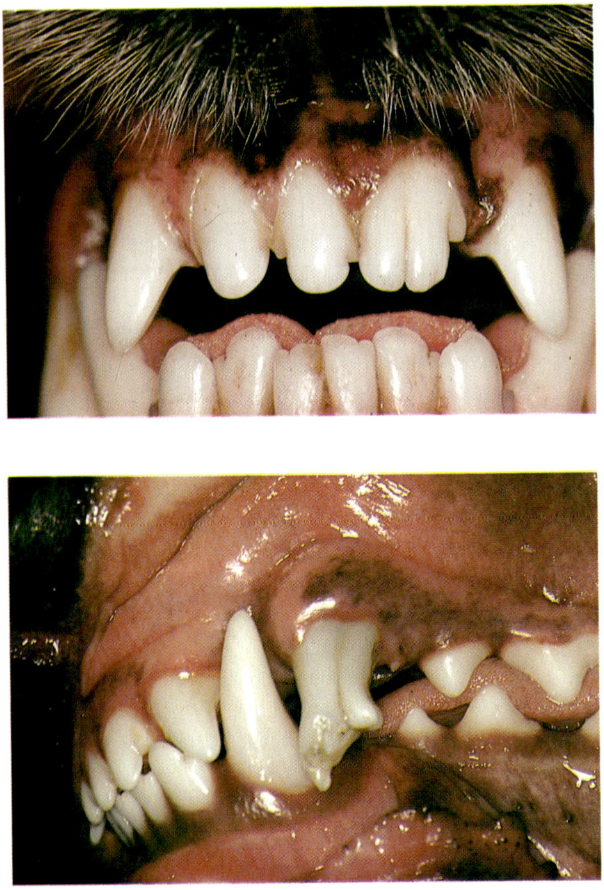

Fig. 4–5. *A*, Twin teeth; *B*, malformed twin canine tooth in a dog.

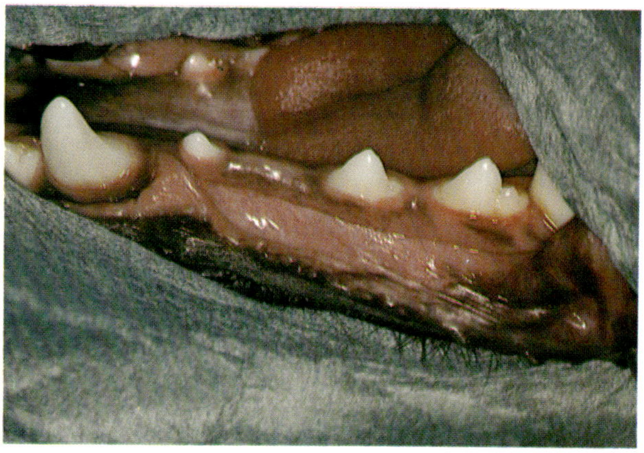

Fig. 4–6. Oligodontia in the mandible of a dog.

Treatment

In herbivores, elongated teeth should repeatedly be ground or cut off; in carnivores, teeth causing trouble should be extracted.

OLIGODONTIA

In certain species of animals, individual or even several deciduous or permanent teeth are not present. In dogs, such teeth often are P1 in both the maxilla and the mandible and the smaller M3 in the mandible (Fig. 4–6).

In the course of change of teeth, the impression of oligodontia may be given by retarded eruption (dentitio tarda), as well as by the traumatic loss of teeth, including loss by extraction.

Some interdental spaces are wider than others, and the alveolar ridge of the jaw at the place of the missing tooth often is narrower than normal and may even be concavely indented. Radiographically, one can trace root portions or, after the third month of life, an unerupted tooth germ. The empty alveolus of a lost tooth can safely be traced up to the fourth week after the loss of the tooth. This fact is especially important when owners of exhibition dogs ask for a veterinarian's certificate that a tooth is missing as a result of trauma rather than of oligodontia. Causes may be missing tooth germs, which in dogs may be hereditary, not the result of lack of space or inadequate use (domestication). The shortening of the jaw, such as in German boxers, leads to a positional change of teeth, but it does not cause oligodontia. In the mandible of brachycephalic breeds of pigs, such as Yorkshires, the distal molar does not erupt, although it does exist.

Not every kind of oligodontia is hereditary, however; tooth germs may also be destroyed by traumatic influences such as infection.

TOOTH RETENTION, DENTITIO DIFFICILIS, IMPACTED TEETH AND PSEUDO-OLIGODONTIA

Occasionally, a patient seems to be missing one or more teeth, or deciduous teeth do not seem to change, although the tooth is visible radiographically (Fig. 4–7).

The impacted tooth usually appears normal in shape and size, but occasionally

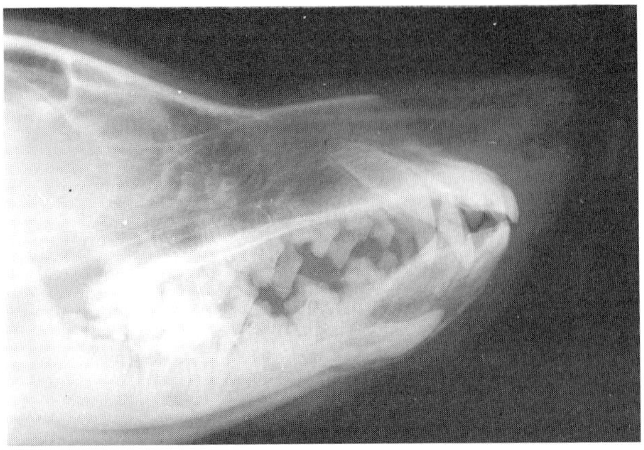

A

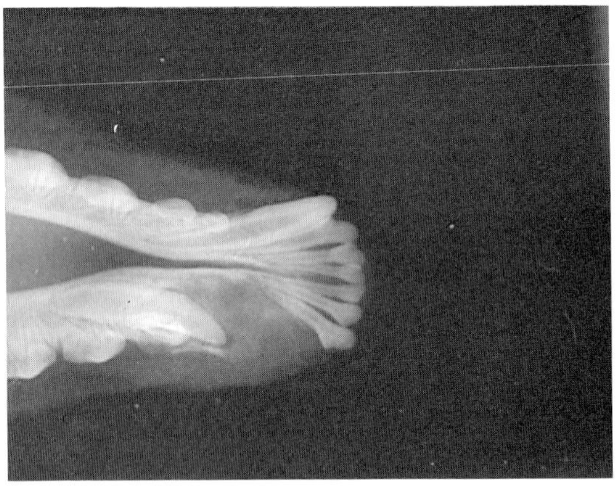

B

Fig. 4–7. *A*, Retention of a canine tooth in the mandible of a dog. *B*, Dorso ventral view.

the tooth germs are malformed and are globular and lumpy or consist of numerous calcified scales separated from each other in toothlike forms. The impacted tooth does not erupt because it grows in the wrong direction or because it is too small to penetrate the gingiva. The already existing, sturdy adjacent teeth are a mechanical hindrance. Externally, vaulting of the gingiva or swelling of the jaw may often be noticed.

Tooth impaction occurs almost regularly with the canine tooth in mares, occasionally with P1 in dogs, and with M3 in brachycephalic pigs.

Treatment

If the tooth crown can be palpated subgingivally, the owner can facilitate eruption by strong massage with the fingertips. Otherwise, the tooth crown has to be exposed surgically with an electrocautery high-frequency surgery unit. Granulation is restricted by astringent fluids or steroidal ointment. When root growth has ended, as determined radiographically, active eruption of the tooth should no longer be expected. Impacted teeth, which cause resorption processes in the jaw or hinder the growth of other teeth, should be exposed and extracted.

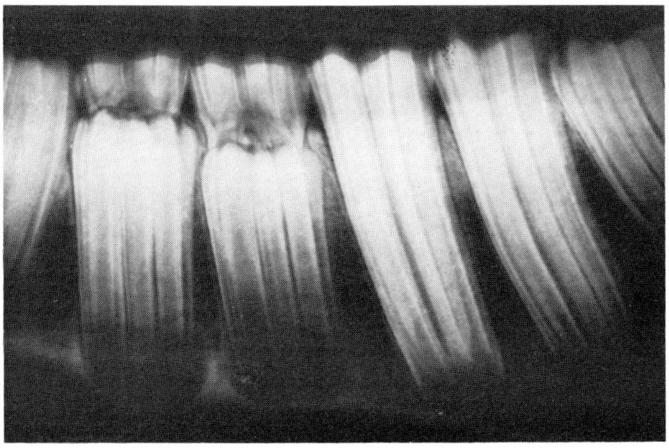

Fig. 4–8. Temporary tooth retention in a horse.

Temporary Tooth Retention in the Horse

In early maturing breeds, a temporary mechanical hindrance of dentition may be the cause of cyst-like swellings in the mandible and of fistulas in the posterior teeth region (Fig. 4–8).

Growth and change of teeth take place earlier in thoroughbreds and in standard breeds than in late-maturing Lipizzaners, Haflingers, and "cold-blooded" breeds of horses. The jaw bones in the foal, especially the arched mandible, are still too short to offer space for all teeth. After the second year of life, M1 and P2 become strong teeth that converge toward the oral cavity; between these, P3 and P4, which are adjacent to M1, have to force their way in. In spite of this occlusal hindrance, tooth growth continues, the rootward pressure of the newly grown tooth tissue causes a hood-shaped, half-round, and limited bone resorption in which the enlarged, yellowish, jelly-like dental sac is situated (Figs. 4–9 and 4–10).

The jaw tries to compensate the reduction of structure by developing a periosteal bony hyperplasia. Symmetric bone swellings become visible at the mandibular margin near the roots of P3 and P4 at the age of 2 years; these swellings disappear when the animal is 5 to 6 years old. The strongly curved M3, which erupts last, often has an enlarged dental sac as well as periapical bone resorption; this strong curvature has its origin in a mechanical hindrance caused by M2. Only the stretched jaw bones in the adult horse offer sufficient space for all posterior teeth.

In unfavorable circumstances, dental fistulas may develop at P3 and P4 and occasionally at M1.

The temporary tooth retention in connection with bone swellings in the mandible heals spontaneously.

DENTAL AND FOLLICULAR CYSTS

Clinically evident symptoms result from the dilatation of a cyst or from secondary bone swelling. The pressure of the cyst causes bone resorption; the cyst wall is often connected with a bony lamella, which consists of bony remnants of the jaw or secondary periostosis of the displaced periodontium or periosteum. This complication occurs frequently with dental cysts that reach into the max-

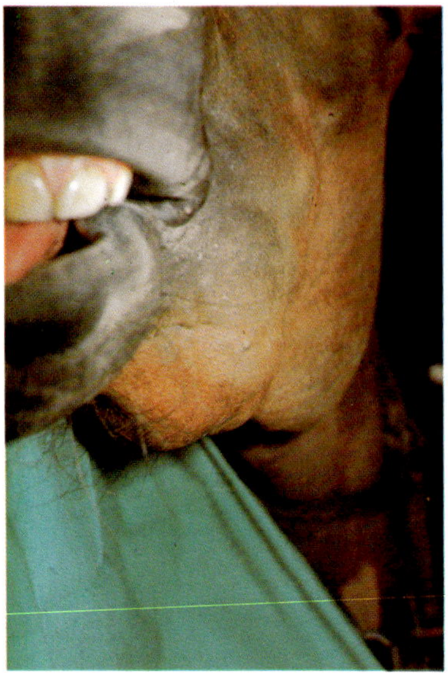

Fig. 4–9. Dental cyst in a 2-year-old thoroughbred. Note the lumpy swelling in the mandible.

illary sinus or the nasal cavity. Unilateral mechanical obstruction of the respiratory ducts, nasal discharge, or empyema may occur in the maxillary sinus that is affected by a dental cyst (horse). The roentgenogram shows hood-shaped or half-globular, limited resorption zones of homogeneous density, often difficult to distinguish in the nasal cavity and maxillary sinus.

The cyst may also contain heterotopic or polyodontal malformed tooth germs (Fig. 4–10).

Follicular cysts may occasionally develop from the enamel epithelium of the tooth crown. Secondary hyperparathyroidism seems to be a common development in dogs and cats. The periapical cysts appear to develop from the em-

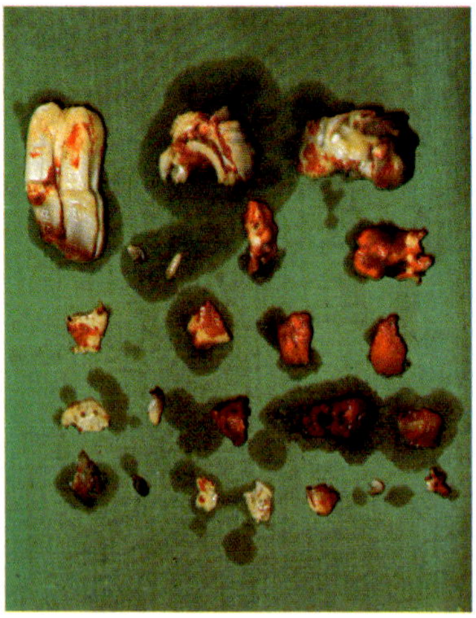

Fig. 4–10. Tooth and tooth fragments removed from the cyst shown in Figure 4–9.

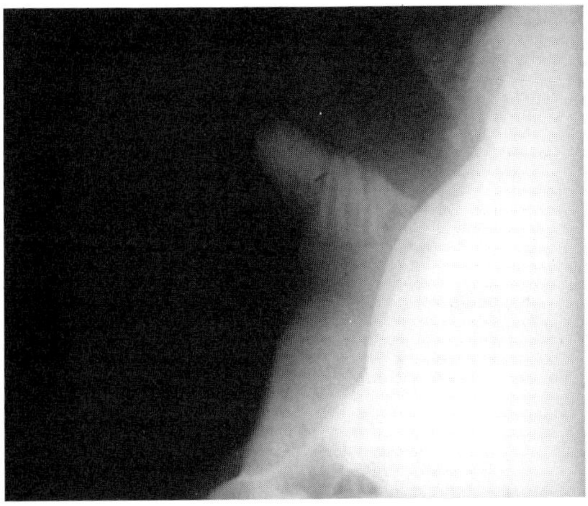

Fig. 4–11. An aberrant tooth in the temporal bone of a horse with an auricular fistula.

bryonal dental epithelium by means of toxic inflammatory irritation, which may result from granulomas at the roots of deciduous teeth.

Treatment

The jaw bone often is thin and should be removed. Another method of treatment is to trephine the nasal cavity or the maxillary sinus. The cyst should be opened; abnormal teeth or tooth germs and, if possible, the whole cyst wall should be removed. When a maxillary sinus has been trephined, the thinly ossified cyst wall will form a cavity separate from the nasal cavity, which contains a yellowing mucous substance and into which an uncovered tooth portion projects. If these portions are malformed tooth germs, they should be removed when possible. The root of a fully functioning tooth should be carefully curetted, and adhering remnants of the cyst should be removed. If the mechanical requirements are met, even a root resection and retrograde filling may be considered.

HETEROTOPIC POLYODONTIA, HETERODONTIA, ABERRANT TEETH, AND AURICULAR FISTULA IN THE HORSE

Either at the jaw or at the skull (temporal bone), one may see a bony swelling that shows no inflammatory processes or promotion in growth.

The auricular fistula in horses, and rarely in sheep, is found at the base of the cranial auricular border at a distance of 2 to 3 cm from the auricle. A mucous liquid flows out of the epithelial opening of the fistula. When exploring with a steel probe, one hits bone or tooth tissue (giving off a peculiar sound) within a few inches. Tooth-like elements of strong x-ray density in the temporal bone can be detected by palpation or, even better, by radiographic examination (Fig. 4–11). Occasionally, a closed, sac-shaped fluctuating swelling is found at the cranial border of the ear. In the cyst or fistula, different epithelial forms such as hairs may often be found.

Cause

Ectodermal tissue, in the form of a branchial cyst or a fistula, originates in the visceral clefts, from which teeth or tooth-like forms develop at a distance from the ectodermal elements. The lesion is identified as a teratoma.

Treatment of Auricular Fistula

A probe should be inserted. Next, a circular dissection of fistula as far as the temporal bone should be accomplished. Loose tooth portions as well as tightly anchored teeth should be extracted. When necessary, sutures should be used. The roots of tightly anchored teeth often are close to the cerebrum, which is easily injured by the forceful extraction of teeth with a chisel.

Displaced teeth that show no clinical reaction need not be treated as long as they do not cause a cyst or fistula. If they do, the cyst wall together with the tooth germ must be completely removed.

HYPOPLASIA AND DISCOLORING

Enamel Hypoplasia in the Dog

Cause

Enamel hypoplasia may be due to lesions occurring during the development of permanent teeth. Because mineralization of tooth crowns in dogs occurs between the fourth and sixth month of life, the disease that causes enamel hypoplasia can be accurately fixed within a given time. In former times canine distemper was thought to be the cause. Any general febrile condition, however, such as intense infestation with worms, pneumonia, gastroenteritis, serious infectious diseases, osteodystrophy, or traumatic lesions, may cause enamel hypoplasia.

Pathogenesis

Edema of the embryonic pulp, or hypoplasia of dentin or of the enamel organ, leads to inadequate or absent mineralization of the hard dental tissue.

Signs and Symptoms

Slight enamel hypoplasia can be recognized by rough, cup-like depressions on the enamel surface. This enamel shows incomplete mineralization and is, in the course of time, subject to strong wear.

Worse enamel hypoplasia can be recognized by enamel defects in the form of points, spots, and circumscribed areas, or those that are linear or hood-shaped. The margin of these lesions usually shows a dark brown discoloration; the exposed dentin has a rough surface and is yellowish brown. Plaque and tartar often develop at these places, but caries are rare. The defects are mostly found on several teeth, but always at exactly the same distance from the gingival margin. The sound enamel covers the crown apices like a hood (Fig. 4–12).

In the differential diagnosis, one should consider abnormal abrasion, such as in fence chewers, tartar, which forms appositions, and caries, which occurs only on individual teeth and in certain locations.

Treatment

Premature abrasion of less-calcified teeth can be prevented by replacing the hypoplastic enamel with fillings or complete crowns.

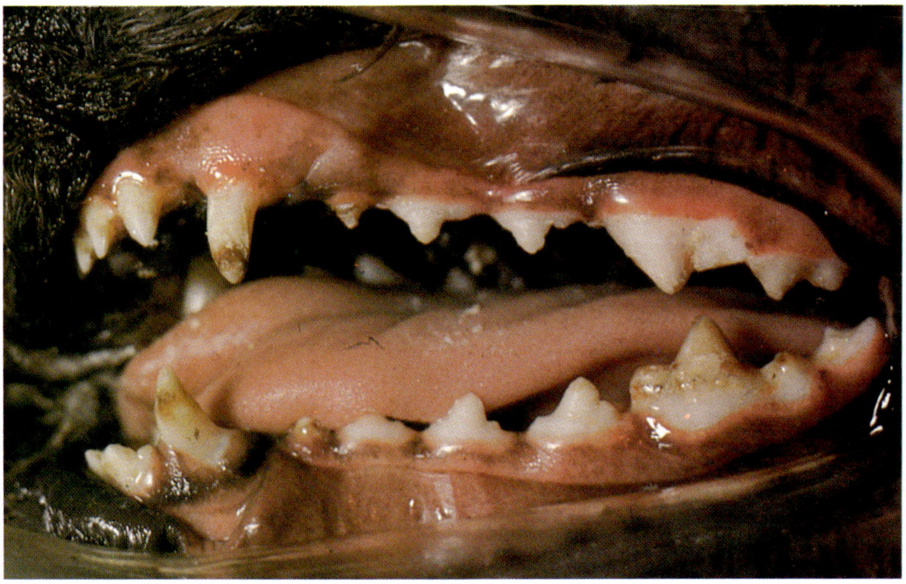

Fig. 4–12. Multiple enamel hypoplasia in a dog.

Minor defects are treated with amalgam or composite fillings. Instructions for cavity preparation should be strictly observed (see Chap. 2); the anchorage of a filling in inferior hard tissue cannot be guaranteed. Major defects at the canines should be repaired with complete crowns of composite material.

Enamel should be ground off; a circular, shallow, semiround cut at the dental neck should be prepared with a rose-head or a pear-head bur (Fig. 4–13).

This technique is ineffective in aggressive, oral-oriented dogs such as guard dogs and fence chewers. The composite material cannot withstand severe occlusal stress. This technique is effective, however, in dogs that are not aggressive chewers.

The preparation must not be too deep; otherwise, the tooth may fracture. Circular and longitudinal channels about 1 mm deep should be cut into the dentin core with a wheel-shaped bur. The surface profile should correspond

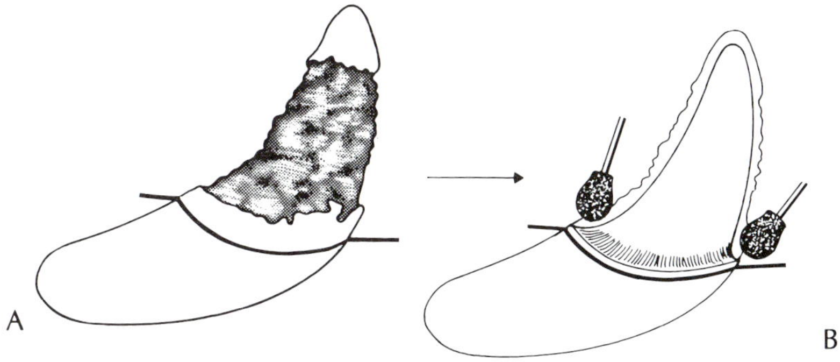

Fig. 4–13. Enamel hypoplasia in a dog: treatment plan. *A*, removal of residual enamel and discolored dental surfaces. *B*, Preparation of a circular, shallow, semiround cut at the dental neck.

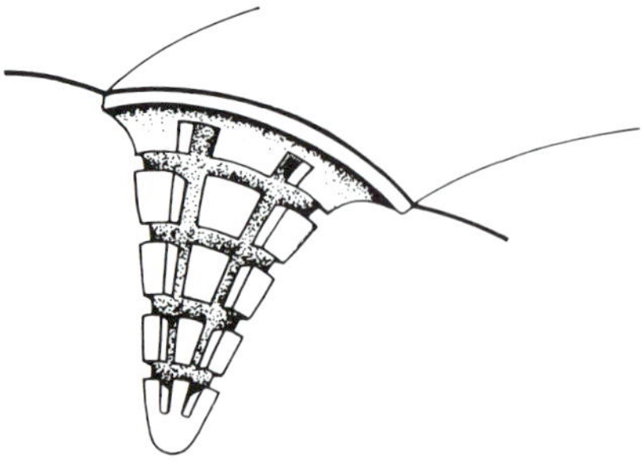

A

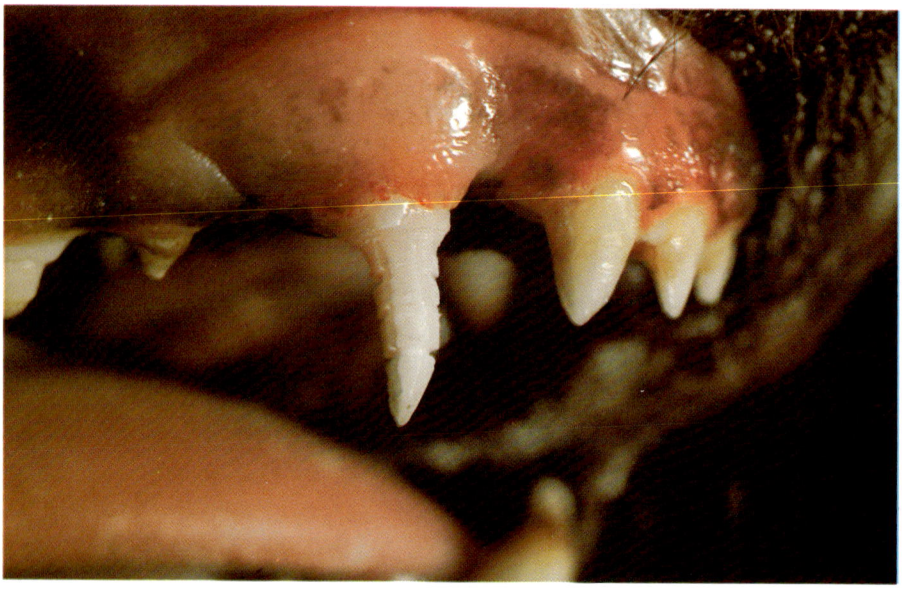

B

Fig. 4–14. Schematic *(A)* and photographic *(B)* views of circular and longitudinal channels in the dentin core (snow-tire tread profile).

roughly to that of a snow-tire tread. This technique gives the composite material adequate mechanical anchorage (Fig. 4–14).

If the distance between the pulp and the surface is less than 2 to 3 mm,—juvenile canines have a wide pulp cavity and thin walls—the dentin tubules should be sealed with a pulp-capping agent such as calcium hydroxide, to prevent the composite material from causing pulpitis.

Composite material in the form of a complete crown is applied to the disinfected and dried surface; this crown can be built up layer by layer with a light viscous material or in one piece with composite paste. In any case, the last layer in multilayered build-ups should have a pasty consistency, so the inorganic filling material guarantees sufficient abrasion resistance.

After hardening, occlusion should be checked and, if necessary, corrected by grinding. If the upper and lower canines are crowded, the crown of the sound antagonist should be ground off so as not to weaken the crown of the tooth under treatment. Final sealing with a glossy sealant, such as Adaptic glaze, is recommended (Fig. 4–15).

Major defects at the sectorial teeth are treated by applying wide, flat fillings,

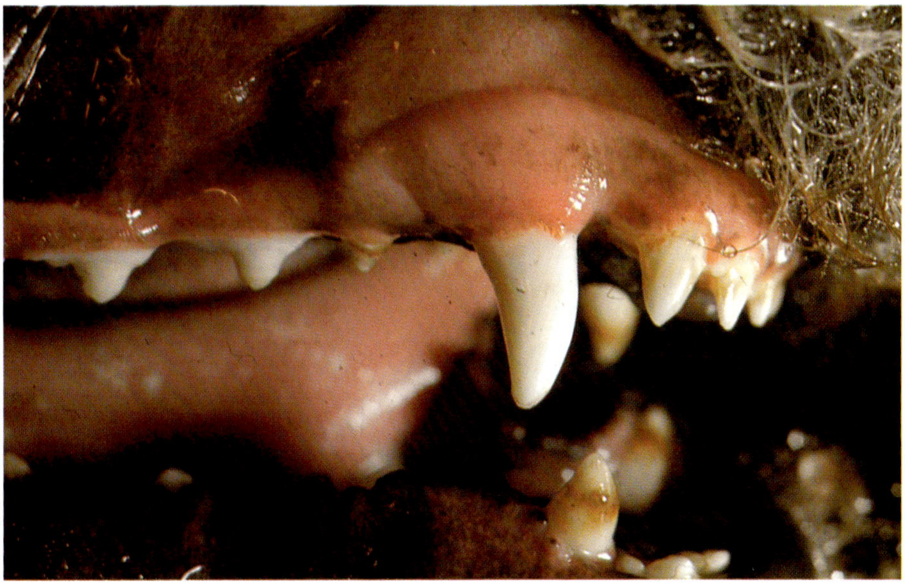

Fig. 4–15. A finished composite crown on a canine tooth after the preparation shown in Figure 4–13.

but only the tooth surfaces need be treated; they are the most used for dissecting the food in the molar region. These surfaces are the buccal surface of M1 in the mandible and the lingual surfaces of both P4 in the maxilla. The cavities extend over the total crowns and are not deeper than 2 mm. In any case, the pulp has to be protected by indirect capping using a liquid agent, such as calcium hydroxide (Fig. 4–16). If a pulp horn is injured during preparation, a vital amputation must be performed (see Chap. 6).

In larger breeds, TMS pins (see Chap. 7) may be used in the tooth center between the pulp horns to guarantee additional strength of the anchored filling.

Amalgam as a filling material is particularly useful because special importance is attached to the border seal of this wide, flat filling, as well as to its anchorage and durability (Fig. 4–17).

Defects on other teeth can be treated with crowns and flat fillings, but modeling and polishing the discolored or cuspal tooth surfaces, especially of less-used teeth (Fig. 4–18), often suffices.

Grinding and Fluoridating. As alternate treatment, grinding off and fluoridating, especially with training dogs, has recently proved useful. Uneven and rough surfaces are ground off and polished until the teeth are white and smooth. When the tooth surfaces are dry, fluoride varnish (Schein Dental Catalog No. 100–0590) is applied; this substance hardens to a sticky yellow coating in 5 minutes. The patient must not be fed for about 10 hours. After this period, when the patient is fed, the varnish will peel away. The dentition will remain smooth, white, and protected against caries for 1 or 2 years. Polishing and fluoridating should then be repeated.

Crown Cement Hypoplasia of Posterior Teeth in the Horse (Fractured Teeth)

For unknown reasons, possibly including systemic disease during dentition or a hereditary defect, the enamel invaginations on one or several posterior teeth

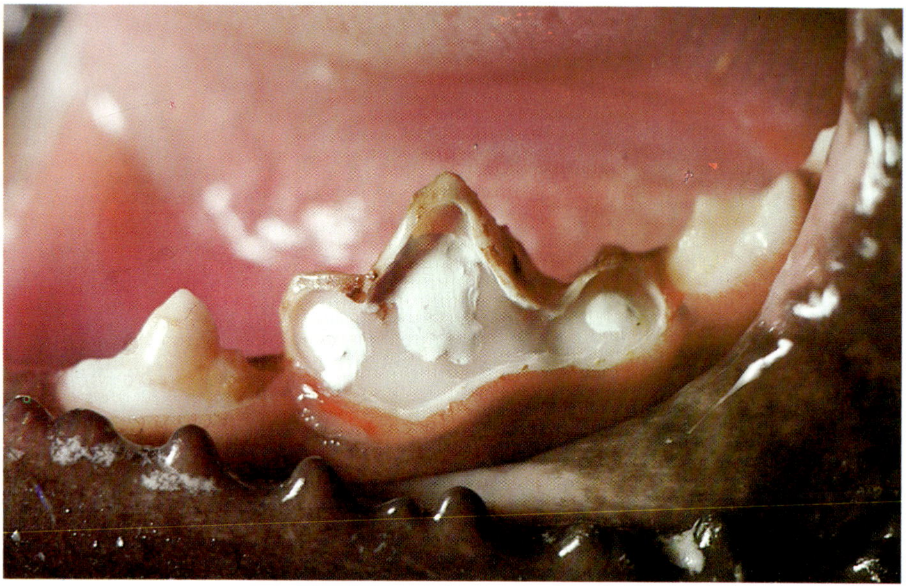

Fig. 4–16. Preparation for shallow filling of a molar. The exposed pulp horns have been covered with pulp caps.

may not be filled with cementum (Fig. 4–19), but the tooth or teeth are not carious.

Food is impacted in the cavities. Because of the swelling of the impacted food and the masticatory pressure, the enamel cylinders break in a longitudinal direction. This process causes pulpitis and alveolar periostitis, but rarely does a

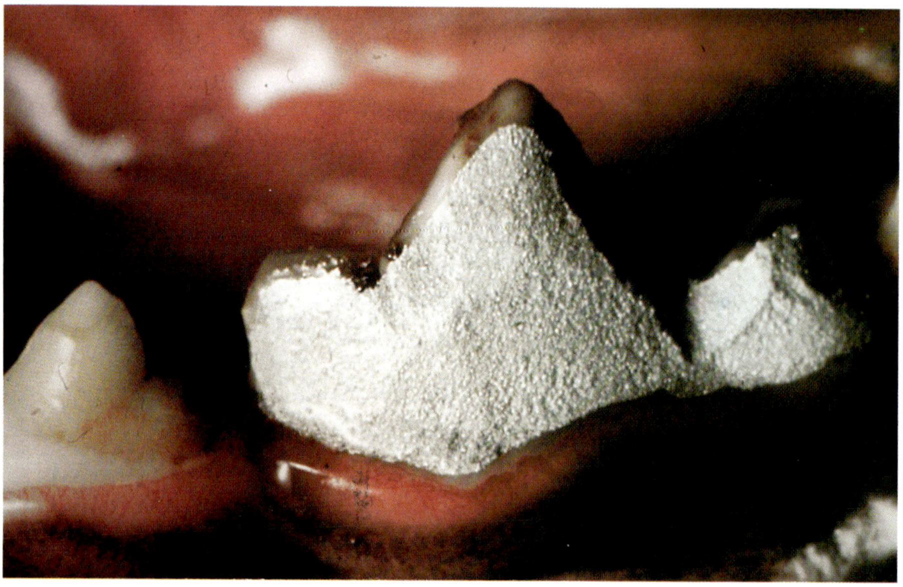

Fig. 4–17. A finished shallow filling, made of silver amalgam, on the tooth shown in Figure 4–16.

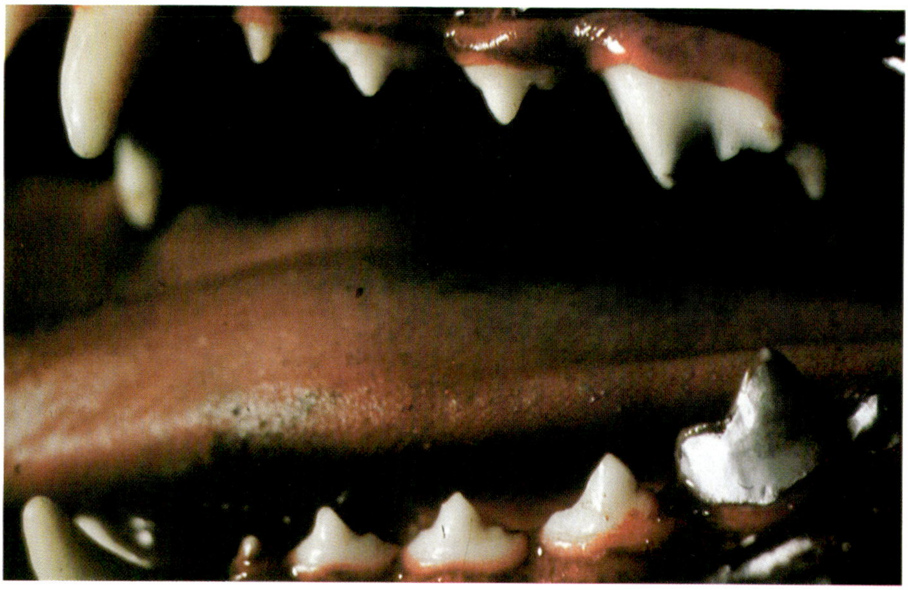

Fig. 4–18. Enamel defect of the canine teeth treated with composite crowns and an enamel defect of the molars treated with shallow silver-amalgam fillings; the premolars and incisors have been polished.

dental fistula form as long as the inflammatory secretion can flow into the oral cavity.

Because the tooth is no longer present, the corresponding tooth in the opposing jaw develops a chisel-like shape (exsuperantia dentis) and causes sore spots.

Treatment

Tooth portions should be extracted, and the protruding antagonist should be ground off; cementum defects can be filled with amalgam, and interdental spaces can be bridged by inlays and anchored with the adjacent teeth.

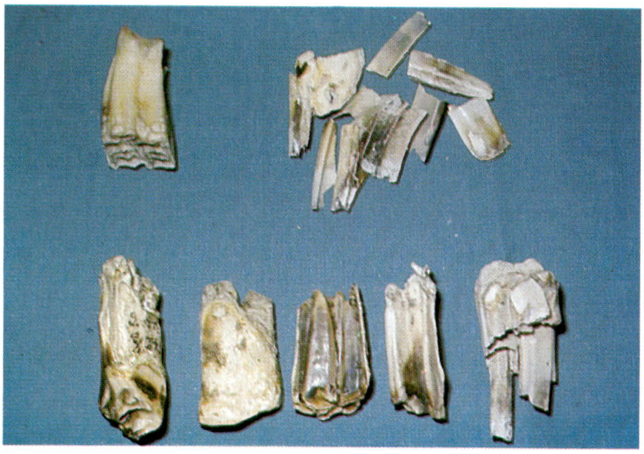

Fig. 4–19. Fractured posterior teeth removed from a horse with crown cement hypoplasia. At the top left is a normally developed posterior tooth.

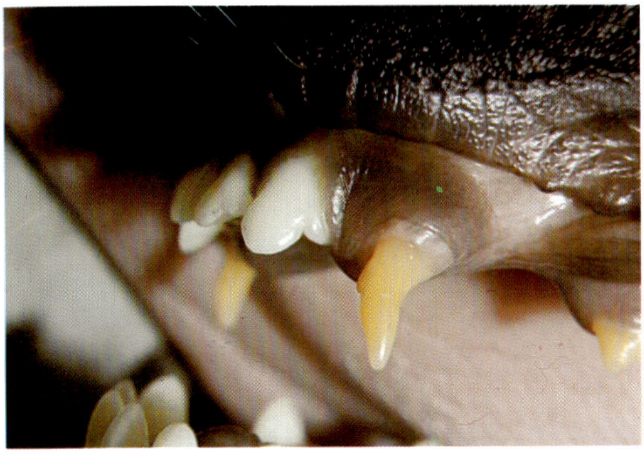

Fig. 4–20. Tetracycline-stained teeth in a dog.

Discolorings

Diseased teeth of small livestock may show a diffusely yellow, grayish, or reddish discoloring when their surfaces remain unchanged. A yellow discoloring indicates a deposition of tetracycline during dentition (Fig. 4–20).

The stain deposits in the bone and hard tooth substance during mineralization. Discoloring is simply an aesthetic disadvantage; to treat, an opaquer, a colored capping of composite material, should be considered.

As a prophylactic measure, tetracycline should not be administered during the first months of life.

Occasionally, a yellowish pigmentation near the gingiva may be seen. This probably depends on food and cannot be removed by the ultrasonic apparatus. A yellowish pigmentation may also result when animals are intensively fed carrots, apples, and pears.

Reddish or rose-colored teeth indicate an existing or an already terminated pulpitis with pulp necrosis (Fig. 4–21*A*).

Erythrocytes extravasate from the pulp capillaries, which have been affected by inflammation or trauma, and invade the dental tubules. Later, the tooth may become grayish because of necrosis and depigmentation. In most cases, the pulp of such teeth becomes necrotic; root canal treatment is therefore recommended (Fig. 4–21*B*).

In horses and ruminants with a sufficient intake of vegetable pigments, such as in carrots, or fruit that is rich in tannic acid, such as pears and apples, a yellow brown, sometimes even dark brown, discoloration may appear in the tooth tissue. This discoloring cannot be removed mechanically.

TUMORS

In most cases, tumors are tissue malformations (teratoidal tumors), caused by developmental disturbances of the odontoblasts.

Ameloblastoma

Ameloblastomas consist of proliferating cells of the embryonic enamel organ, but they can develop from remnants of the epithelial sheath of the periodontal membrane, the so-called epithelial sheath of Malassez, in later years. They have

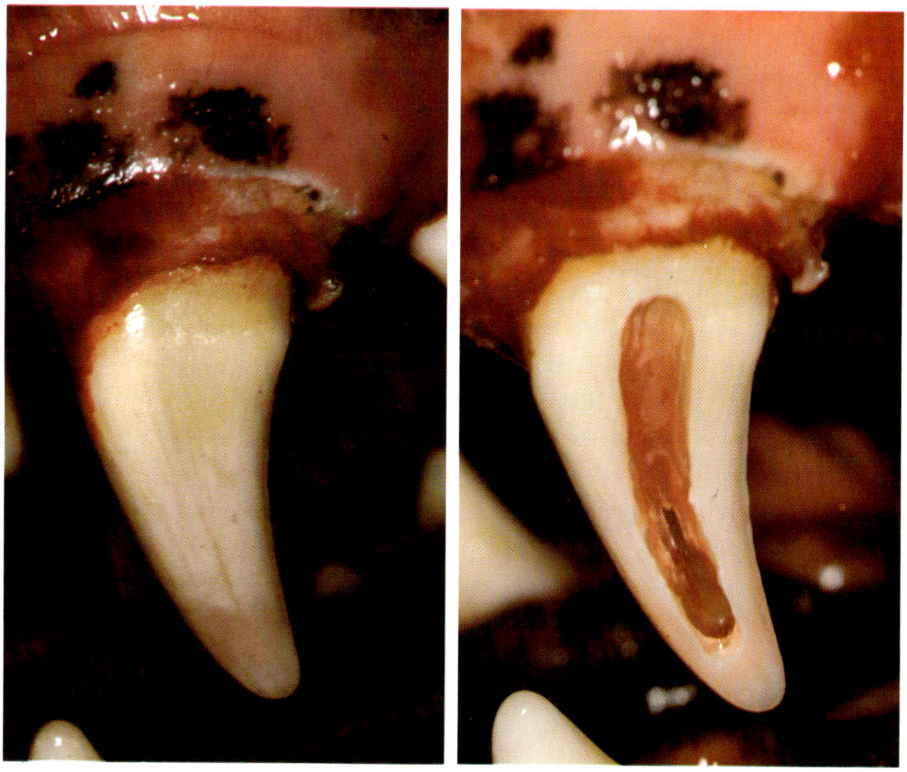

A B

Fig. 4–21. *A*, Reddish discoloration of a canine tooth in a dog (pulpitis). *B*, After the removal of surface layers, the blood-filled dentin canals become visible. The pulp canal, opened in the coronal region, is full of dark brown residual pulp.

only sporadically cartilaginous, calcified enamel deposits and can therefore be cut; they are occasionally interspersed with cysts. Ameloblastomas expand rapidly and may recur if portions of the tumor are left after an operation. Pressure atrophy and periosteal bone growth cause round cavities; adjacent teeth are loosened and displaced. The lumpy masses of tissue, which proliferate toward the oral cavity, are covered by a mucous membrane, which is often ulcerated.

Ameloblastomas in cattle are occasionally found in the incisor region of the mandible, but rarely at other locations or in other animals. In most cases, total extirpation of a large ameloblastoma fails because of its tendency to spread into the cavities of the altered jaw bone. Change into a true carcinoma has occurred.

Odontoma

Odontomas are neoplasms of the abnormally proliferated dental papilla; in addition to dentin, they contain both enamel and cementum (Fig. 4–22).

If the tissue remains at a slightly differentiated embryonal state, a soft, dental-like *minor odontoma* is produced. If hard tooth substances are produced, a *hard odontoma* develops. The *odontoma simplex* may originate from a tooth of normal dentition and regular position, from a displaced but erupted tooth, from a supernumerary tooth (polyodontia), or from an impacted tooth germ. This kind of odontoma can deform the tooth to an irregular shape; often only the crown

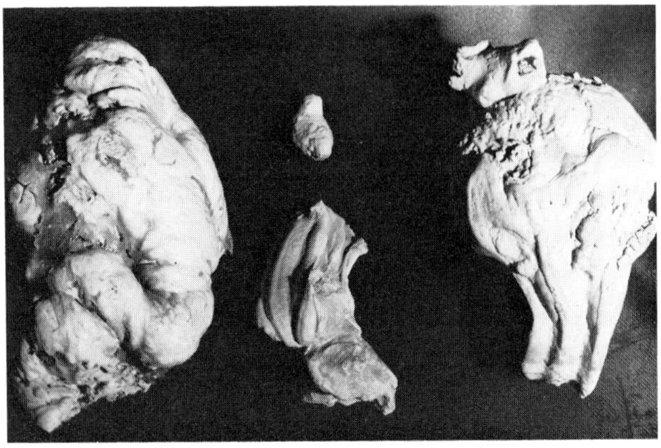

Fig. 4–22. Odontomas removed from horses.

or the root of the tooth is deformed. In horses, and rarely in cattle, these tumors occur as coronal odontomas at the posterior teeth or incisors. They have a dental-like hard consistency, are the size of a fist, and are lumpy. They usually do not continue growing in the postembryonic stage of development, and they do not metastasize. Smaller odontomas, therefore, can be removed surgically. Root odontomas mostly consist only of dentin and cementum.

The *odontoma multidentiferum proliferans* originates from either one multifractured tooth or from several tooth germs. It may belong to the normal row of teeth, but it may be polyodontal as well. It consists of numerous, sometimes hundreds, of small, rudimentary, dental-like forms; its tissue cells continue splitting and growing after the animal is born. The odontoma multidentiferum proliferans is benign and does not metastasize although tumor cells that remain postoperatively cause the tumor to recur. It is always connected with an alveolus and may cause bony exostosis and penetrate into the maxilla and the nasal cavity. Occasionally, this form of odontoma can be seen in horses and cattle 1 to 3 years old.

Cementoma

The cementoma is a limited, tumor-like cemental thickening at the crown or root of an otherwise normal tooth. It develops during embryonic growth and may continue growing in the postembryonic stage of development by cemental apposition if it is at the interalveolar part of the tooth. A cementoma is different from inflammatory local cemental hyperplasia, which, like bony exostosis, develops as a result of a periodontitis.

The grayish white cementoma has a hard consistency; it often cannot be clinically distinguished from an odontoma. Intra-alveolar odontomas or cementomas may complicate tooth extraction.

Bibliography: 2, 3, 4, 5, 11, 12, 13, 20, 47, 58

5

Orthodontics

Orthodontics is the branch of dentistry involving the repositioning of malplaced teeth. Most animals have an anisognathous dentition; that is, the maxilla is wider than the mandible, which often is slightly shorter as well.

NORMAL OCCLUSION IN THE DOG (DOLICHOCEPHALIC SKULL)

Incisor Region

These animals have shear mouth; that is, the mandibular incisors are in minimal contact with the lingual surfaces of the maxillary incisors. The mandibular canine tooth is in an occlusal position and equidistant between I3 and C in the maxilla.

Posterior Teeth

The maxillary P4 articulates with the mandibular M1. The sectorial cusp of the mandibular M1 engages between the maxillary P4 and M1. In occlusal position, the crowns of the mandibular molars are mesial in the interdental space of the corresponding maxillary premolar. The distal buccal cusp of the mandibular M1 articulates with the central pit of the maxillary M1. This tooth position is called *orthognathous molar relation.*

Premolar Occlusion

The peaks of the crowns of the mandibular premolars insert directly into the diastema of the maxillary premolars.

Dental Planes

The maxillary and mandibular arches are parallel when the mouth is closed.

ABBERATIONS FROM NORMAL JAW FORM

Mesial Occlusion

The mandible is longer than the maxilla (Fig. 5–1). Other terms for this kind of occlusion are mandibular prognathism (see Fig. 5–11), prenormal occlusion, and undershot jaw (in horses). True mesial occlusion is rare. All mandibular

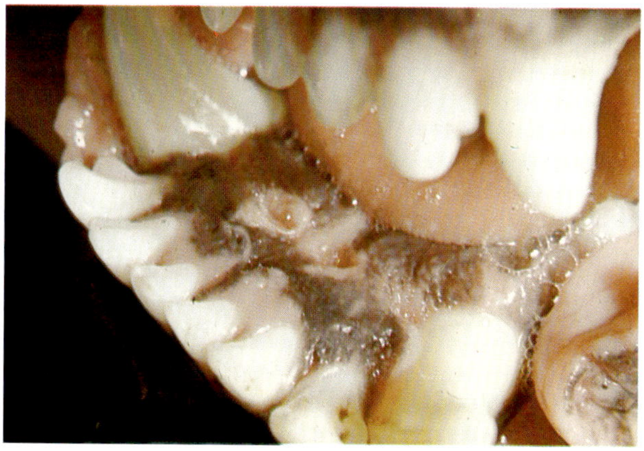

Fig. 5–1. Mesial occlusion. The maxillary incisors have produced pressure necrosis in the mandibular gingiva.

posterior teeth, including the molars, have been displaced forward by a half or even full tooth width (displaced molar relation).

The apparent mesial occlusion shows a normal molar relation; the incisors, and often the premolars as well, project too far forward. The diastema of the premolars is wider than usual. This configuration is typical for brachycephalic breeds of dogs, such as boxers and bulldogs, but it is an aberration in dolichocephalic breeds. The maxillary incisors may cause painful pressure necrosis in the gingiva of the mandible. Particularly unfavorable conditions exist in rodents, in which the continually growing incisors may become abnormally elongated from lack of abrasion.

Distal Occlusion

The mandible is shorter than the maxilla. Other terms for this kind of occlusion are maxillary prognathism, overshot jaw, and parrot mouth (in horses—Fig. 5–2). It also occurs in dogs with long, pointed noses, such as miniature dachshounds, Italian greyhounds, and collies (Fig. 5–3).

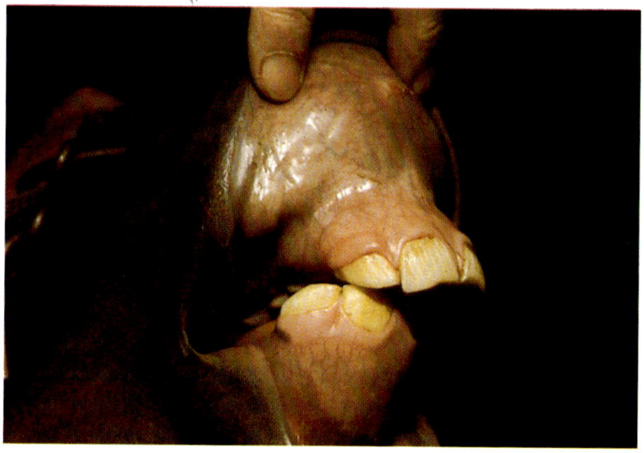

Fig. 5–2. Distal occlusion (parrot mouth) in a horse.

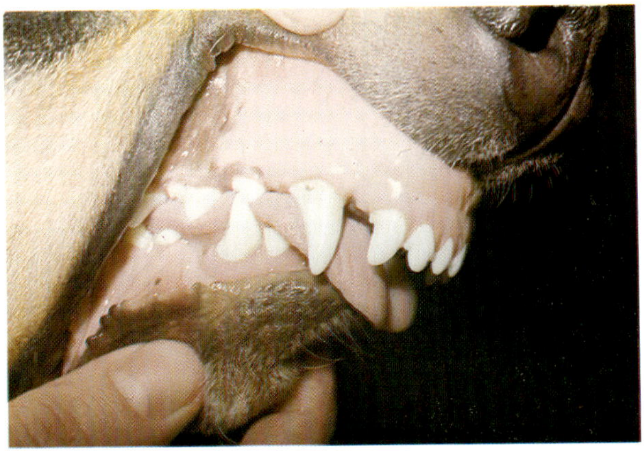

Fig. 5–3. Distal occlusion in a dog.

The mandibular incisors, and even the canines in cases of tooth crowding, cause gingival lesions in the maxilla. A displacement of molar relation in horses entails only a partial abrasion of the maxillary P2 and often of the mandibular M3 as well. Hook-shaped apophyses are formed.

ABERRANT TOOTH POSITION

Irregular Dental Row (Crowding)

The incisors are not in line, but rather are irregular in their arrangement and position in the dental row (Fig. 5–4).

Tooth Crowding

The canines, mostly those in the maxilla, are crowded and injure the soft parts of the opposing jaw (Figs. 5–5 and 5–9).

Crossbite

In half the incisor region, shear occlusion is present, and in the other half, inverted incisor distance is seen (Fig. 5–6).

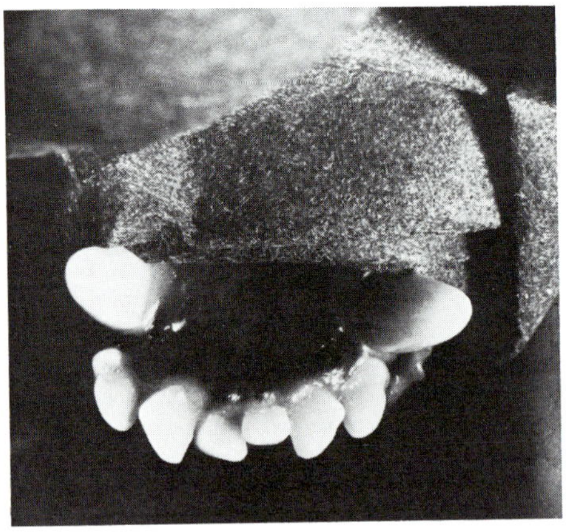

Fig. 5–4. Irregular dental row (crowding) in the mandible of a dog.

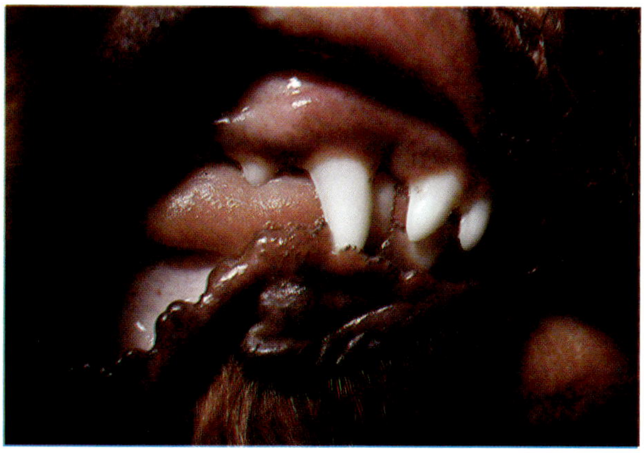

Fig. 5–5. Tooth crowding of the mandibular canine teeth in a dog.

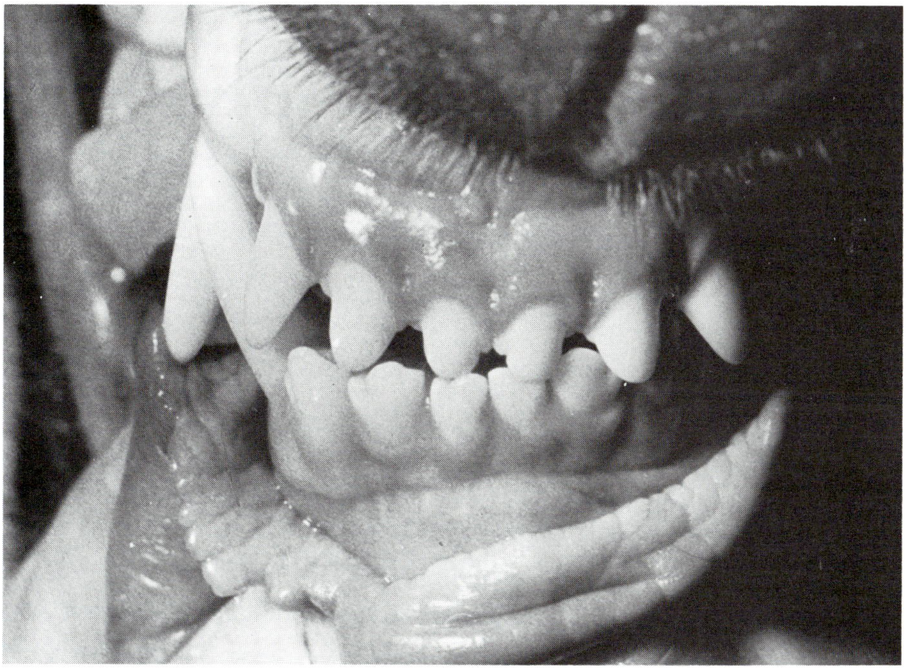

Fig. 5–6. Crossbite in a dog.

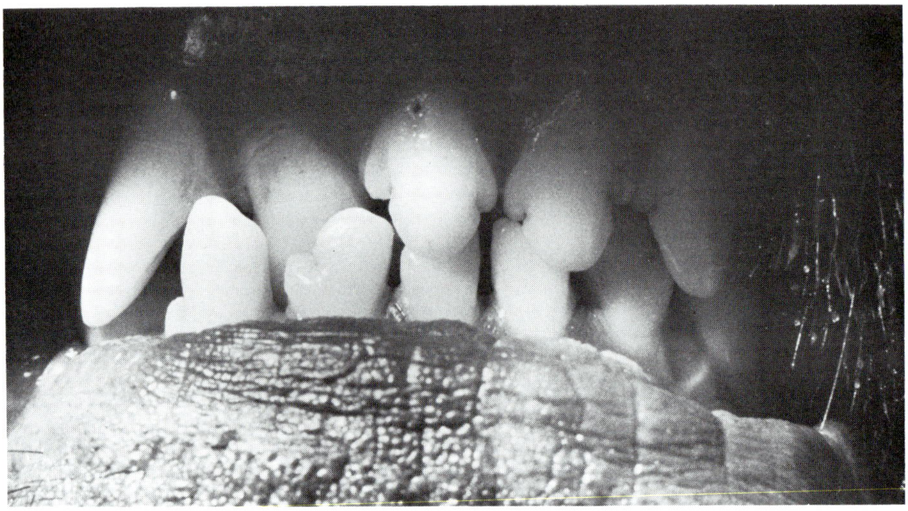

Fig. 5–7. Malrelation of individual teeth; retrusion of the I2 in the right side of the maxilla.

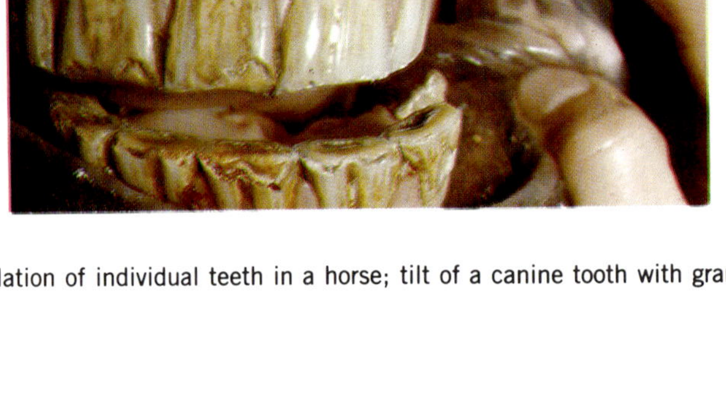

Fig. 5–8. Malrelation of individual teeth in a horse; tilt of a canine tooth with granuloma in the lip mucosa.

Malrelation of Individual Teeth

Common malrelations are protrusion, retrusion (Fig. 5–7), torsion, and tilting or lateral deviation (Fig. 5–8).

CAUSES OF MALPOSITION OF TEETH AND JAWS

Genetic Causes

The mode of inheritance is still unknown. A polygenic factor is likely and may take effect after one or more generations.

Mechanical Causes

Such causes include congenital trauma or traumogenic injury before or during dentition and alveolar and jaw fracture.

Deciduous Tooth Persistence

The permanent canine appears to be displaced laterally.

CLINICAL IMPORTANCE OF MALPOSITIONS

An otherwise sound, well-cared-for dentition may show asymmetric abrasion. Premature loss of teeth may be caused by a liability to periodontosis, for example, as in breeds of miniature dogs such as poodles and dachshunds. Because of missing antagonists, such teeth may become abnormally elongated. Other possible causes include injury to soft parts, cellulitis, osteomyelitis, and difficulty with food intake. Some or all of the foregoing causes may lead to periodontitis.

TREATMENT

Orthodontic treatment has, so far, only been applied to incisors and canines in dogs. Canine-crowding correction should be performed at the age of 7 to 10 months, but correction of the incisor arch should not take place before age 10 to 12 months because the canines are used as abutment teeth for the orthodontic appliance and should therefore be firmly anchored in their sockets. A correction could also be effected at a later date. Canine crowding and moderate mesial and distal occlusion are simple to correct.

Bilateral Canine Crowding (Figs. 5–5 and 5–9)

Treatment should start when 5% of the canine tooth has erupted. A sturdy encased expansion screw, suitable for the canine distance, is cemented onto the canine with composite by means of an acid-etch technique (see Chap. 7). In small breeds, encased screws (see Chap. 2), which are cemented on directly, suffice.

In large breeds of dogs, Biederman's expansion screw is useful. The projecting wire ends are curved into a ring or a half-ring on the plaster model or, if necessary, directly on the patient's teeth. They are then slid over the canines and cemented onto them (Fig. 5–10).

Before positioning, the screw should be loosened so it can slide over the divergently projecting canines up to the base of the crown. Occlusion should be checked.

The screw should be activated every 4 to 6 days by inserting the pin in the spindle and turning it once by 90°. In this way, the screw halves are moved

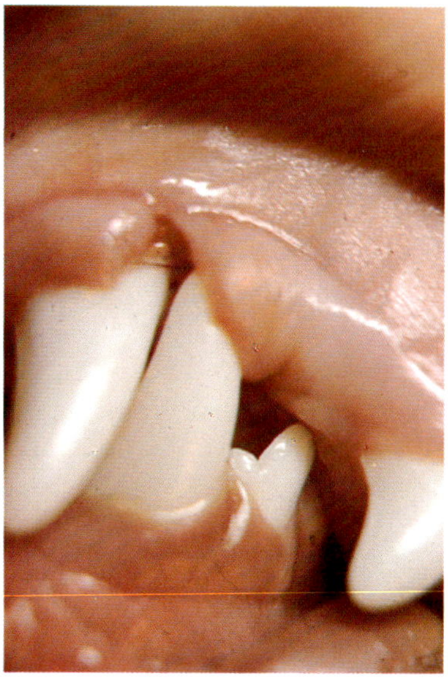

Fig. 5–9. Tooth crowding of canine teeth and distal bite in a dog. The maxillary gingiva is injured.

away from each other by 0.25 mm. It is easier for animals to tolerate this kind of adjustment when, in the first days of treatment, oral tranquilizers are administered. Average treatment time, when activating is done in intervals from 4 to 6 days, is 2 to 4 months. Once the orthognathic tooth position has been achieved, the screw must remain in its final position for some time. The position of the appliance should repeatedly be checked because the screw may turn back by itself. Fixation time is approximately equal to activating time.

If teeth are not fixed long enough in their final position, recurrence of the malformation is likely.

In many cases, the screw should be removed and replaced by a suitable piece of steel wire; this wire is then fixed onto the teeth, which by now should be in the right position. The wire is then cemented onto the teeth by means of the enamel etch technique. The patient does not experience so much discomfort with the wire as with the screw.

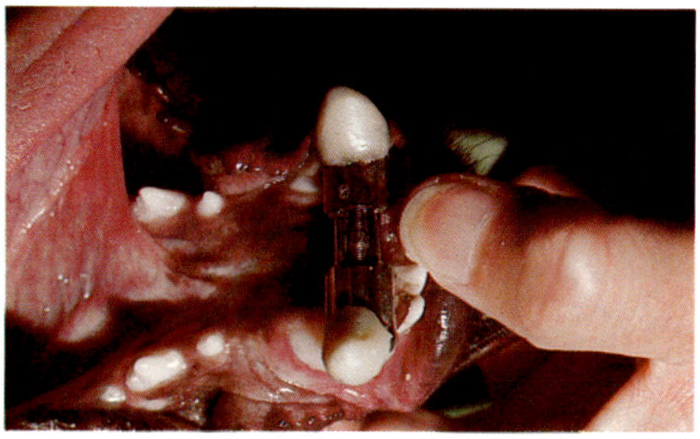

Fig. 5–10. Treatment of canine tooth crowding. An expansion screw has been cemented onto the canines by the enamel etch technique.

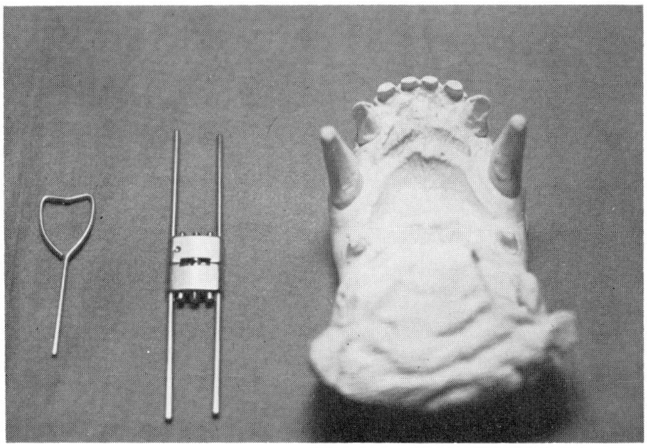

Fig. 5–11. Hyrax expansion screw with pin and plaster model.

The screw is removed by milling off the composite. Below the regulating screw, plaque may cause gingivitis, which heals within a short time.

Regulating the Incisor Arch

The American Kennel Club and most veterinarians consider orthodontic therapy unethical when efforts are made to camouflage genetic malocclusions. Although all animals are entitled to healthy occlusion, not all are entitled to perfect occlusion. Because the majority of requests for orthodontics in "show dogs" deals with an anterior crossbite of the incisors, particular attention must be paid to the total occlusal relationships of all teeth. Any deviation from normal of the canine, premolar, or molar occlusion in these dogs suggests a genetic cause and precludes orthodontic therapy. If only the incisors are involved and if all other occlusal parameters are normal, however, then trauma is suspected, and orthodontic therapy should be instituted.

Protrusion

An expansion screw on the model is embedded in acrylate to form a bar between the canines (Figs. 5–11 and 5–12). Acrylate is a mixture of powder and

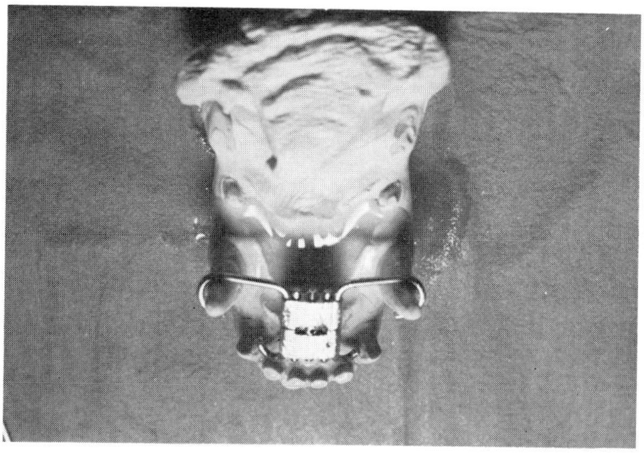

Fig. 5–12. Adjusting the wire ends to a plaster model.

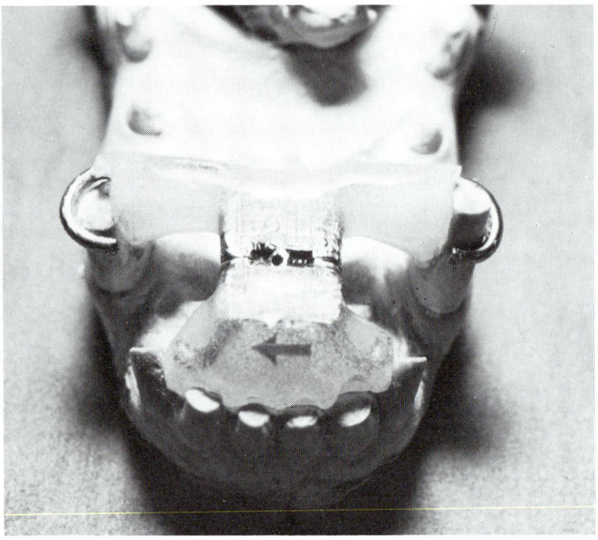

Fig. 5–13. Embedding the wire ends in acrylate. The arrow indicates the direction in which to turn the spindle.

a liquid; its consistency depends on individual requirements. A fluid mixture readily flows into the channels and indentations of expansion screws. The mixture should be viscous or even pasty if a special shape is to be formed, such as a bar on the anteriorly protruding parts (Fig. 5–13).

Molding on the model can be done manually; the material keeps its plasticity for up to 10 minutes and then hardens gradually. A preceding coating with an isolating agent prevents the acrylate and the model from sticking together. One drop of acrylate on the hardening surface smoothes any unevenness and saves subsequent grinding and polishing operations.

Acrylate is adapted to the oral part of the screw in such a way that it not only connects with the anterior part of the screw, but also ties close to the posterior

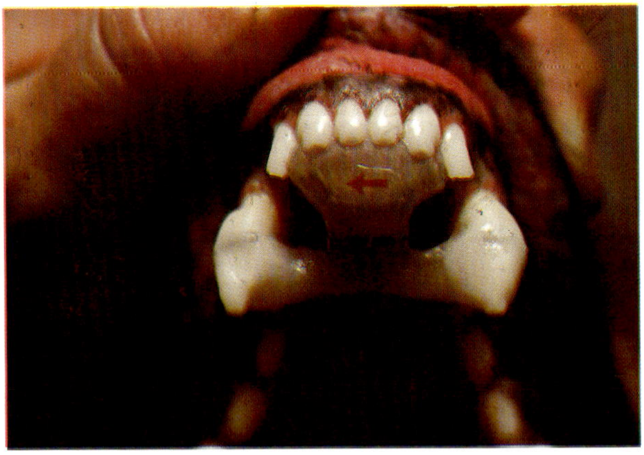

Fig. 5–14. Orthodontic device (arrow) cemented onto the canines.

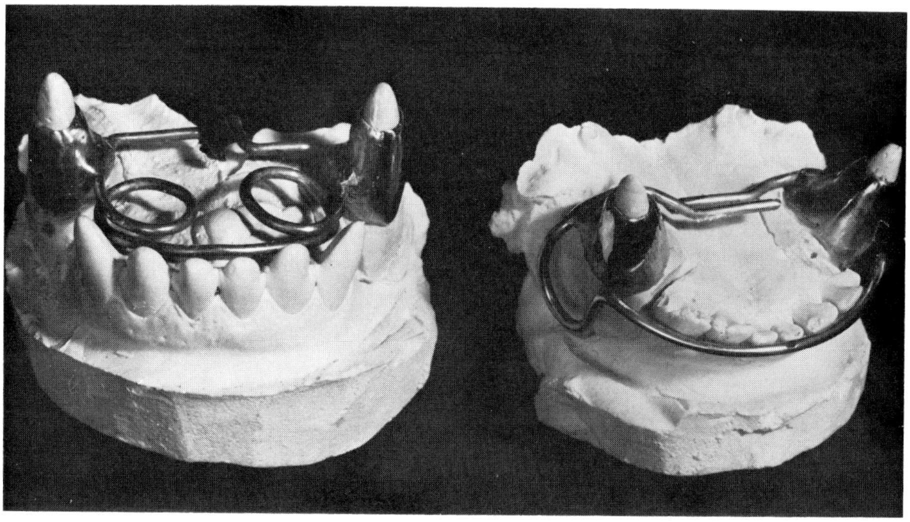

A B

Fig. 5–15. Orthodontic devices with activating loops on plaster models.

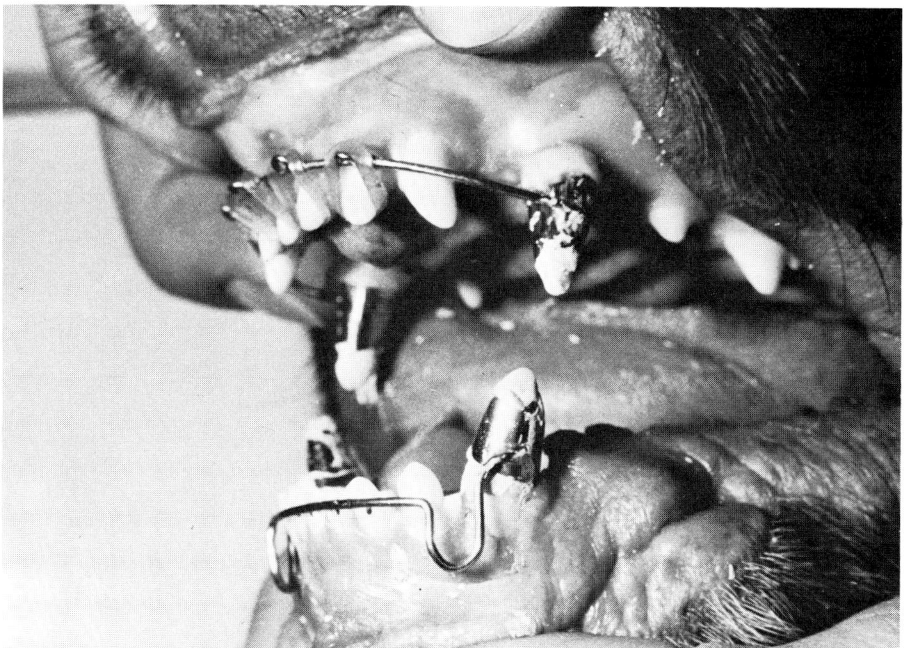

Fig. 5–16. Protrusion of maxillary incisors by rubber rings; retrusion of mandibular incisors by the labial arch with an activating bow.

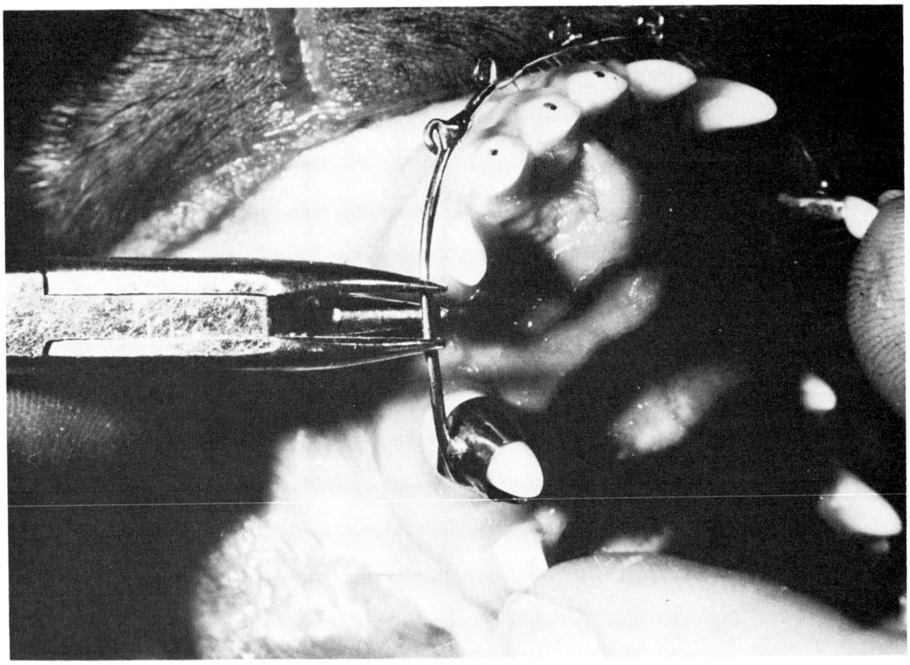

Fig. 5–17. Activating the labial arch with pliers.

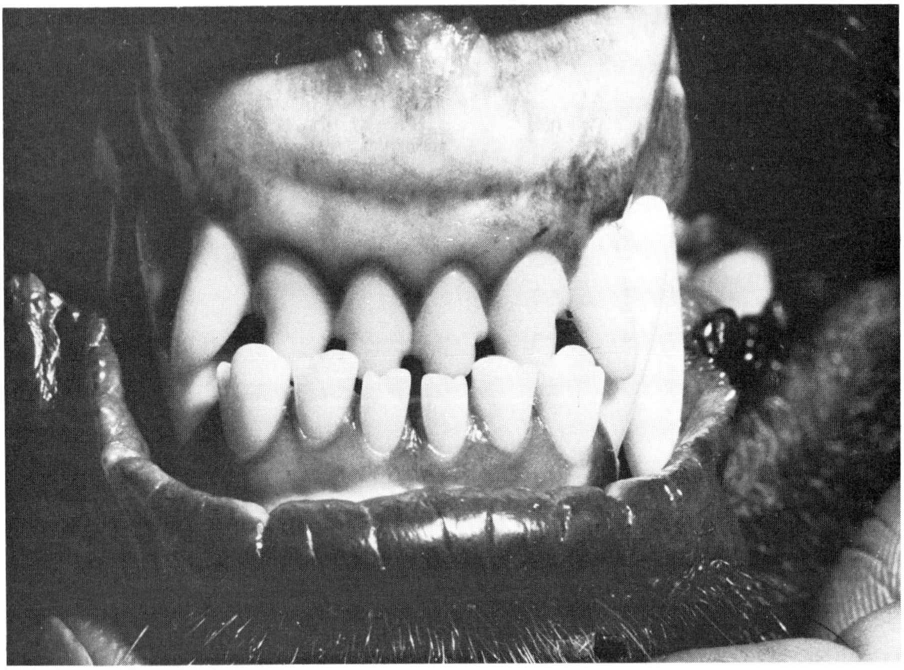

Fig. 5–18. Superior brachygnathia in a dog.

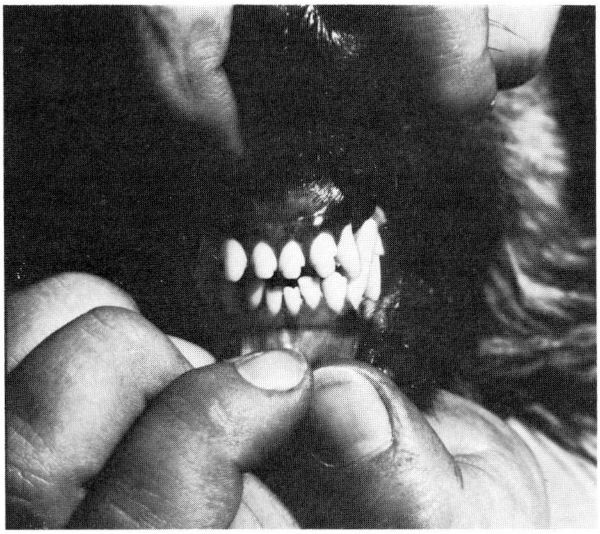

Fig. 5–19. Successful treatment maintains orthognathic incisor distance.

surfaces of the incisors. The apparatus is then ready to be cemented onto the canines (Fig. 5–14).

In the event that individual incisors protrude more than others, the anteriorly protruding portion of the appliance must lie close to them. At first, however, the appliance may be farther from the incisors that are less protruded. In some cases, the anterior part of the expansion screw must be prevented from sliding off the curved lingual incisor surfaces by creating a step to counteract it (Fig. 5–15). This step should be neither sharp nor too deep; otherwise, the tooth or teeth may fracture.

Retrusion

The simplest way of regulating retrusion is by means of a labial arch with two activating bows (Figs. 5–15 and 5–16). A pair of Aderer pliers is used to form the activating bows. The labial arch can be applied by means of bands or partial crowns on the teeth, or it can be cemented directly onto the enamel. The labial arch is activated by contracting the wire bow with Aderer pliers (Fig. 5–17).

The arch exerts pressure on the incisors from the front and thus moves them aborally (Figs. 5–18 and 5–19). The labial arch must be made of heavy wire, or it may be bent by the patient.

Regulating Individual Teeth

Individual teeth are regulated by activating loops (Fig. 5–20) or with sturdy, encased expansion screws in acrylate. Forming the model is easier when the acrylate is mixed until it is viscous. The anterior part of the encased expansion screw lies close to the tooth and moves it after activating.

The orthodontic appliance is cemented onto the abutment teeth (in most cases, the canines) with adhesive composite. An arrow indicates the direction in which the owner should turn the spindle.

Transparent plastic forms can be added to the model with vacuum adaptors

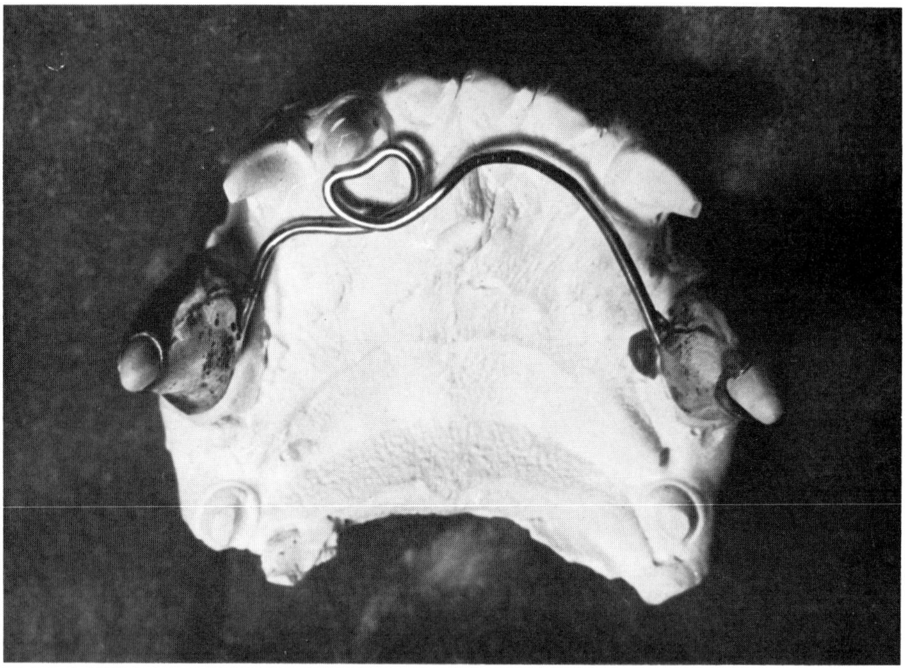

A

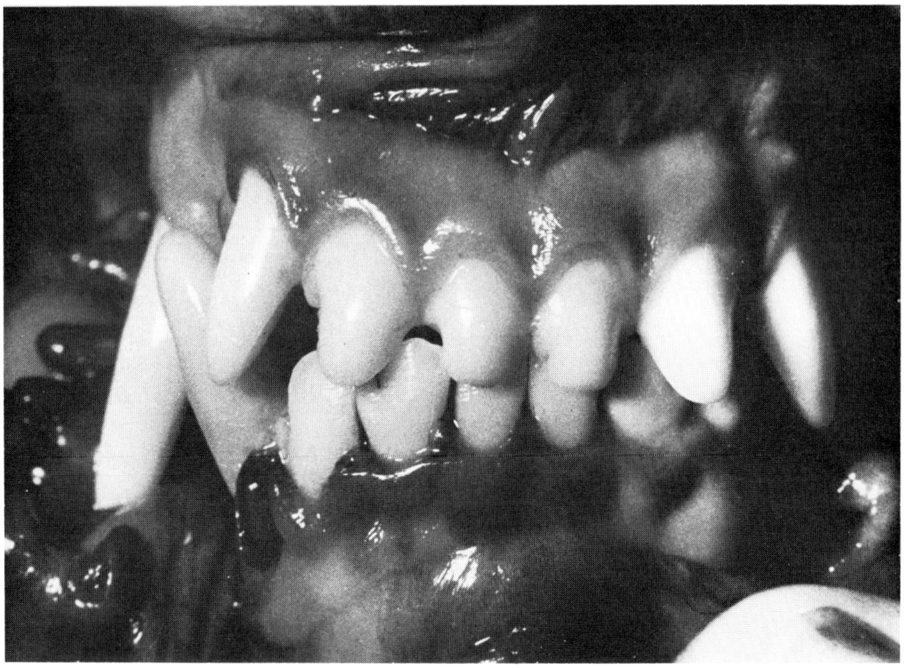

B

Fig. 5–20. *A,* Activating loop for protrusion of an incisor. *B,* Successful treatment 8 weeks later.

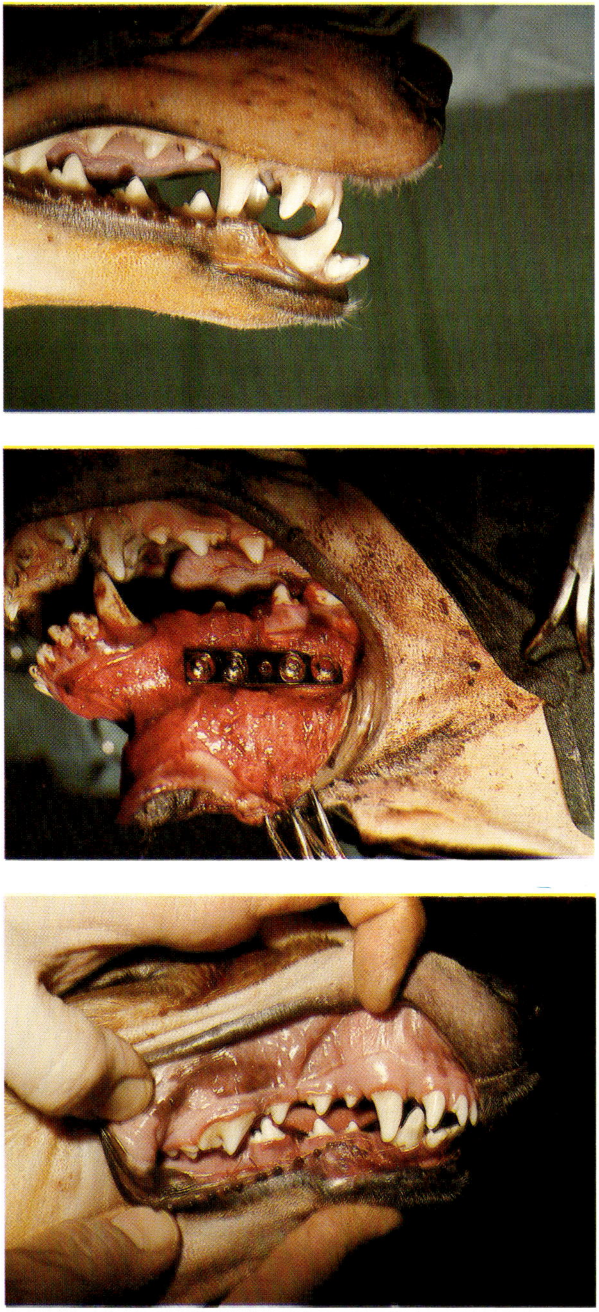

A

B

C

Fig. 5–21. *A,* Mesial occlusion in a collie. *B,* Partial jaw resection with application of a jaw plate. *C,* Successful treatment 6 months after operation.

and specially shaped anterior parts rather than with manually molded bars. The regulating elements of the appliance are embedded in these transparent forms; these forms correspond exactly to the teeth onto which they are cemented. Thus, one avoids the unwanted moving or drifting of abutment teeth that often occurs with simple appliances. A disadvantage is the cost of the vacuum adaptor. We recommend that dental clinics that have no specially trained personnel have such models made by dental laboratories.

A particular malposition, common in the mandible of dogs, is the overlapping of M1 by P4, which may occur in either arch. In this malocclusion, the small last mandibular premolar is placed too distally and too posteriorly and partially covers the mesial part of the crown of P1. Because self-cleaning is impossible in this part of the dentition, food debris, hair, and plaque readily collect. As a result, tartar, especially subgingival tartar, periodontitis, root caries, and difficulty in eating may develop.

Treatment

The distal cusp of P4 should be ground off. If this procedure exposes the pulp, then amputation of the distal root of P4 and pulp-cap therapy of the mesial root should be done under sterile conditions. A simpler solution, however, is total extraction of P4, thus salvaging the more important M1. Plaque can be thereby removed, and self-cleaning is made possible. When required, tartar removal, gingivectomy, and odontoplasty may be performed (see Chap. 9). Extremely malformed jaws can only be treated surgically by osteotomy and the application of eccentric dynamic compression plates. According to our experience, the procedure, which requires cutting the mandibular canal, including the arteries, veins, and nerves passing through it, is clinically irrelevant (Fig. 5–21).

Bibliography: 3, 5, 23, 43, 45, 48, 50, 62, 64

6

Tooth Fracture and Alveolar Fracture

TOOTH FRACTURE NOT INVOLVING THE PULP

Minor enamel lesions and superficial tooth fractures that do not expose the pulp are found often in dogs and occasionally in horses. Tooth fracture may be caused by trauma, such as from biting hard objects.

Signs and Symptoms

Tooth fractures appear as sharp-edged dental defects. They have a rough, dim, yellowish surface and may be sensitive to temperature at first. The rough surface enhances the formation of tartar and plaque. If the lesion reaches as far as the pulp, which then shines through with a rose color, pulpitis may develop in reaction to bacterial and chemical irritations or thermal changes.

Treatment

Sharp points should be ground off. The exposed dentin tubules, in which the sensitive prolongations of the odontoblasts are contained, should be sealed with indirect pulp-capping agents, such as calcium hydroxide. For this purpose, the lesion is coated, if necessary more often than once, with dentin sealants or, in case no sealant is at hand, with a 5 to 10% silver nitrate solution. Major lesions may be coated with acid-etch bonded composite. Occlusal defects in herbivores gradually disappear as a result of normal abrasion.

TOOTH FRACTURE EXPOSING THE PULP

Oblique, transverse, and comminuted fractures are likely to be found at the enamel cusps in carnivores as well as at the incisors and canines in herbivores (Fig. 6–1).

The enamel folds of posterior teeth in herbivores usually fracture longitudinally, often exposing the alveolus. Tooth fractures in dogs primarily affect the canines and the upper sectorial tooth; tooth fractures in herbivores affect the

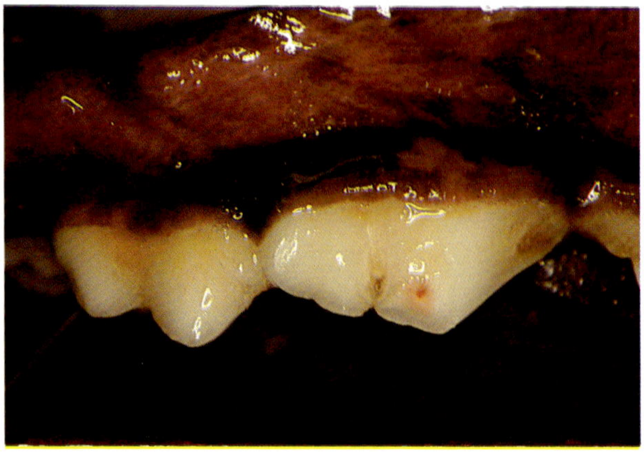

Fig. 6–1. Recent tooth fracture of a P4 in a dog.

posterior teeth. The pulp can also be exposed by excessive shortening of the teeth; such as by grinding of the canines in domesticated animals, or by large-scale caries treatment.

Any injury to the pulp causes pulpitis. The pulp tissue is not only mechanically injured by trauma, but also is chemically affected by the toxicity of the oral flora. Such influences may gradually affect the entire pulp. Rarely does the pulp have enough resistance to survive in spite of the trauma. This is particularly striking in the growing teeth of herbivores and the continuously growing teeth of rodents.

Recent Pulp Exposure

Pulp exposed by traumatic injury or surgical operation bleeds strongly in the first few minutes, but a vital pulp exposed for a longer time retracts into the root canal. The opening of the root canal is filled with a dark brown plug that consists of food debris and bacteria (see Fig. 6–4).

It is important that the pulp of juvenile teeth be kept vital before the roots have fully developed, to guarantee normal dentition and dentin formation. The wide root opening also offers unfavorable preconditions for mortal amputations and root fillings.

Treatment

Indirect Pulp Capping. If the pulp is visible through a thin layer of dentin, the application of dentin sealants, such as calcium hydroxide, will protect the pulp from noxious irritations and will stimulate the formation of secondary dentin (Fig. 6–2*A*).

Direct Pulp Capping. If the pulp is exposed during a dental procedure, such as deep carious or shallow fillings on sectorial teeth in animals with enamel hypoplasia, a small amount of any calcium hydroxide capping agent, following application of a hemostatic substance such as epinephrine or hydrogen peroxide, is applied to the exposed pulp with a cotton pellet without exerting any pressure; a thin coat of pulp-protection cement is then applied (Fig. 6–2*B*). The cavity may be sealed temporarily and should be checked for inflammation or infection in 8 to 10 days. These complications are uncommon; as a rule, a temporary

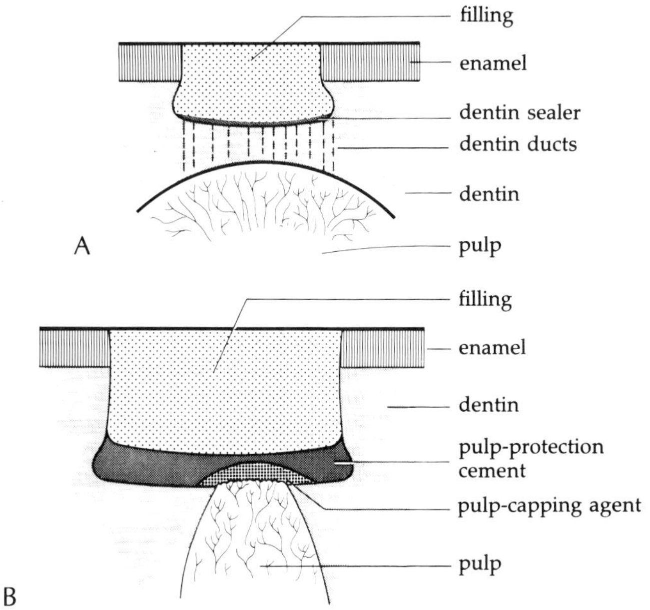

Fig. 6–2. *A*, Schematic view of indirect pulp capping; *B*, schematic view of direct pulp capping (see also Fig. 4–16).

filling is not necessary, and a permanent filling of amalgam or composite can be inserted. The traumatized pulp heals because of the antibacterial and anti-inflammatory effects of the capping agents; calcium hydroxide enhances the formation of secondary dentin. Any pulp exposure lasting more than 8 hours must be considered old and contaminated. If the direct pulp-capping technique is used, antibiotic therapy is indicated. Because most apical granulomas require up to 6 months to develop, intraoral radiography is indicated 6 months post-operatively to establish the absence of abscess formation, indicating continued pulp vitality.

Vital Amputation. Even in a recent tooth fracture, the pulp tissue is superficially infected. Some 3 to 4 mm of the pulp must therefore be removed with a handpiece (Fig. 6–3*A* and *B*). The interior of the cavity is conically prepared with an inverted cone bur or a pear-shaped bur, to ensure the retention of later fillings (Fig. 6–3*C*). A hemostatic substance, such as epinephrine or hydrogen peroxide, is applied. Without exerting any pressure, one then applies a capping agent to the pulp with a cotton pellet.

Steroid-containing capping agents must be used with caution because they reduce resistance to infection and may lead to pulp necrosis in spite of antibiotic protection. The best capping agents are calcium hydroxide preparations, which have a pH-neutralizing and anti-inflammatory effect for a long period of time.

Pulp-protection cement is applied to the layer of calcium hydroxide with an instrument that fits the size of the defect without exerting pressure. Permanent sealing is done with amalgam or composite (Fig. 6–3*D*).

Older Tooth Fractures with Infected Pulp Necrosis

Single-rooted teeth in carnivores are treated by extirpating the necrotic pulp and filling the root (Fig. 6–4).

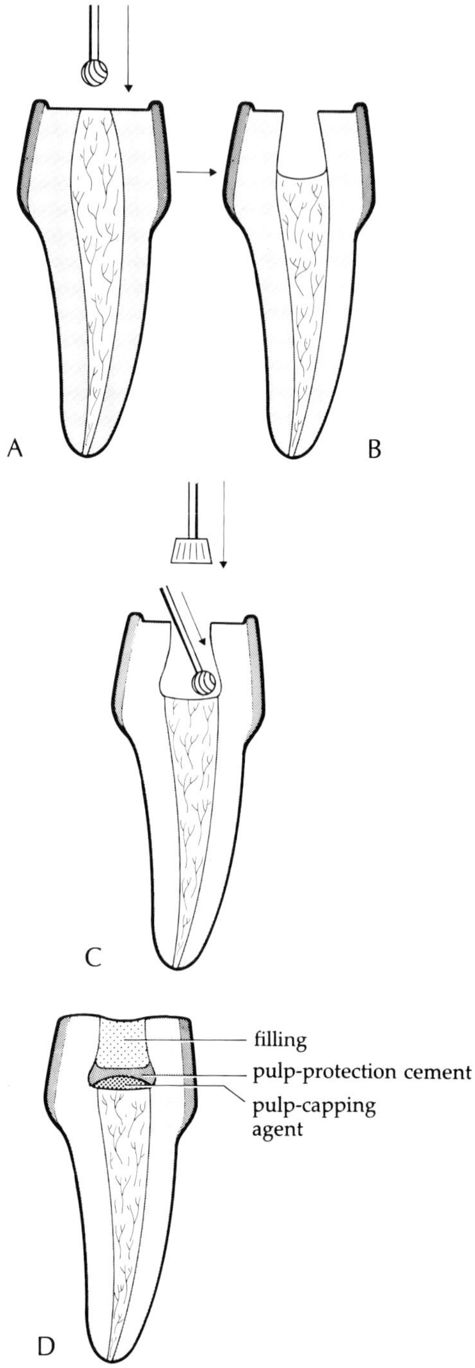

Fig. 6–3. Schematic view of vital amputation. *A,* Tooth before treatment. *B,* Removal of superficially injured pulp. *C,* Inverted conical enlargement of cavity; rounding of sharp dentin edges with a rose-head bur. *D,* Sealing of the cavity in layers with pulp-capping agents, pulp-protection cement, and filling.

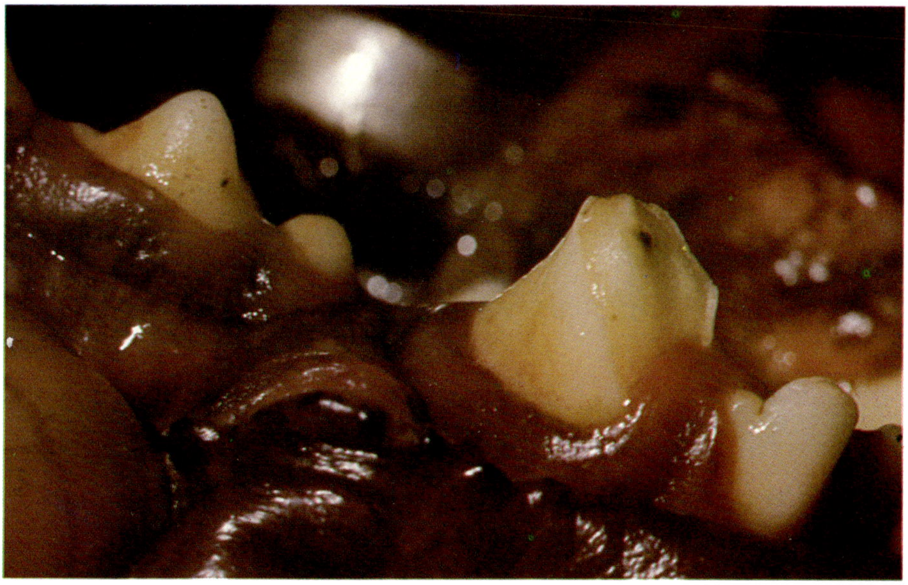

Fig. 6–4. Old fracture of a canine tooth in a dog. The root canal opening is visible as a dark spot.

Recently erupted permanent teeth must be treated with utmost care because of their wide root openings. Multirooted teeth, particularly those with curved roots, may make instrumentation and complete filling of the root canals difficult. An alternate treatment, especially for less-experienced practitioners, is mortal amputation, which has been modified for veterinary purposes and can be performed in one visit (Fig. 6–5*A*).

A few weeks later, a clinical and roentgenographic follow-up should be scheduled, to examine the patient for a possible apical granuloma.

With mortal amputation, as much of the reachable pulp tissue as possible is removed (Fig. 6–5*B*); the tooth is then rinsed with a disinfectant solution. Some Formocresol is applied to the pulp stump, and the cavity is permanently filled (Fig. 6–5*C*).

Formocresol is a strong disinfectant that mummifies and disinfects the residual pulp. If bacteria survive the disinfectant, a periapical granuloma or a dental fistula may develop later.

As a rule, any fractured deciduous tooth with exposed pulp should be extracted. Because of the position of the permanent tooth bud, apical abscess formation of the deciduous tooth puts the permanent tooth at risk for developmental defects. Endodontic therapy is usually difficult to complete successfully on deciduous teeth. Moreover, because the deciduous teeth remain in the animal's mouth such a short time, extraction of the affected teeth is the easiest way to resolve the problem.

Pulp Extirpation

If the pulp has been severely traumatized from a tooth fracture, or if an infection has rendered it necrotic, the residual pulp must be extirpated (Fig. 6–6). The exposed pulp cavity, often filled by debris, can be seen as a brown or black small opening on the fractured surface (see Fig. 6–4).

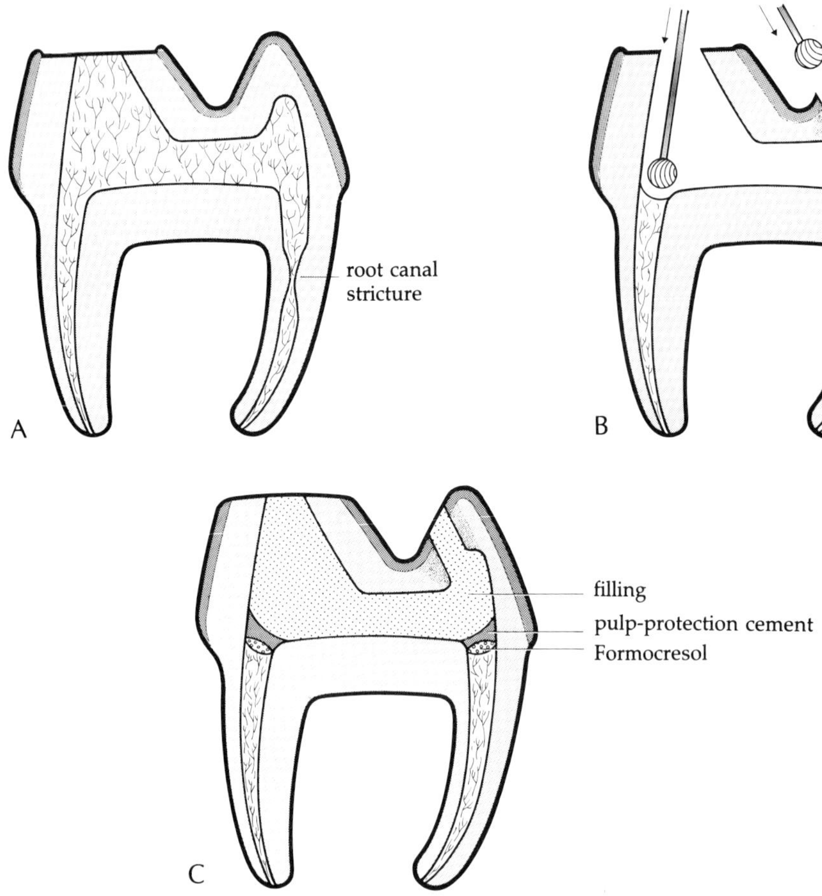

Fig. 6–5. *A,* Indication for mortal amputation: multirooted teeth with strongly curved roots and constriction of the root canal. *B,* Schematic view of mortal amputation, with removal of the reachable pulp. *C,* Sealing with Formocresol in layers; protective cement filling and permanent filling of cavity.

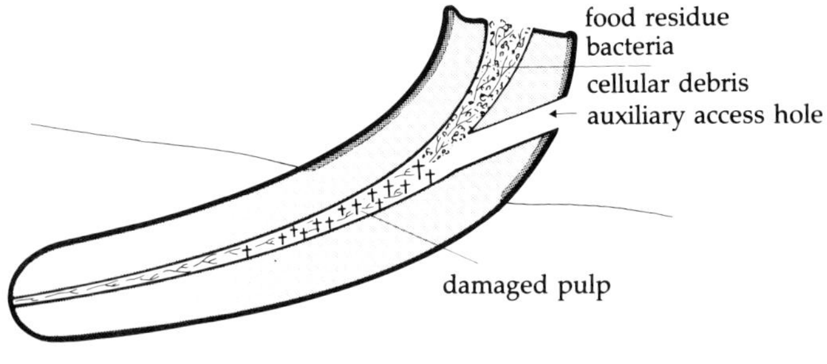

Fig. 6–6. Indication for pulp extirpation: strongly traumatized pulp or excessive pulp necrosis. One gains access to the root apex by an auxiliary hole because of the strongly curved root.

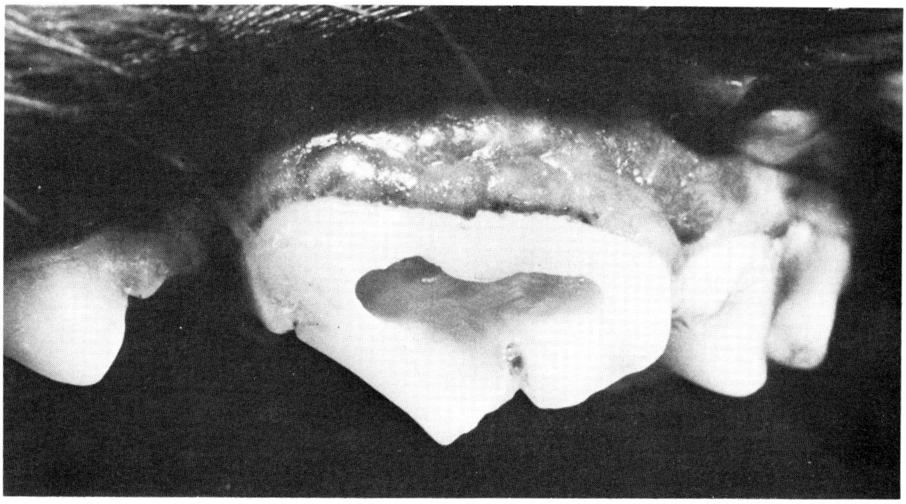

Fig. 6–7. Presentation of the root canal entrance of a multirooted tooth that is ready for extirpation of the pulp.

For pulp extirpation of a canine tooth, an auxiliary access hole above the gingiva is necessary (Fig. 6–6). The pulp cavity of multirooted teeth must be exposed sufficiently to enable one to see the root canal entrance (Fig. 6–7).

In extirpating the pulp, one inserts a barbed broach into the nerve canal; as one slowly turns the barbed broach, the pulp is threaded onto it (Fig. 6–8*A*). The barbed broach, together with the pulp, is then carefully pulled out of the root canal (Fig. 6–8*B*). In many cases, the pulp is necrotic, so only dark brown debris catches on the broach.

When the pulp has been extirpated, the root canal should be rinsed with a disinfectant solution, such as alcohol. The root canal should then be cleansed chemically with hypochlorite and then neutralized with a 3% hydrogen peroxide solution. A final rinse with saline solution is recommended. These preparations are applied to the root canal with a small-gauge needle.

Once it has been disinfected and cleansed, the pulp cavity should be dried by air and paper points. The subsequent mechanical preparation of the root canal by filing ensures the removal of infected dentin layers (Fig. 6–9).

The pulp canal should be rounded off with root-canal files by starting with the smallest size and then by using successively larger files; filing can be done manually or mechanically (Giromatic-angle handpiece, see Chap. 3). One should continue filing until the chips of dentin are dry and white; then one should rinse with a disinfectant and dry with an air blower or paper points.

Care must be taken to remove all necrotic debris from the root canal to the apex of the tooth. Intracranial radiographs with the files inside the canal help one to determine the length of the tooth as well as the working length of file to be used. Care must be taken to avoid driving the tip of the file through the apex of the tooth. Teeth that have been broken for many years have severe lysis of the apex. Consequently, the opening of the apical foramen is the size of the root canal. This distorted anatomic feature makes it easy to violate the apex by

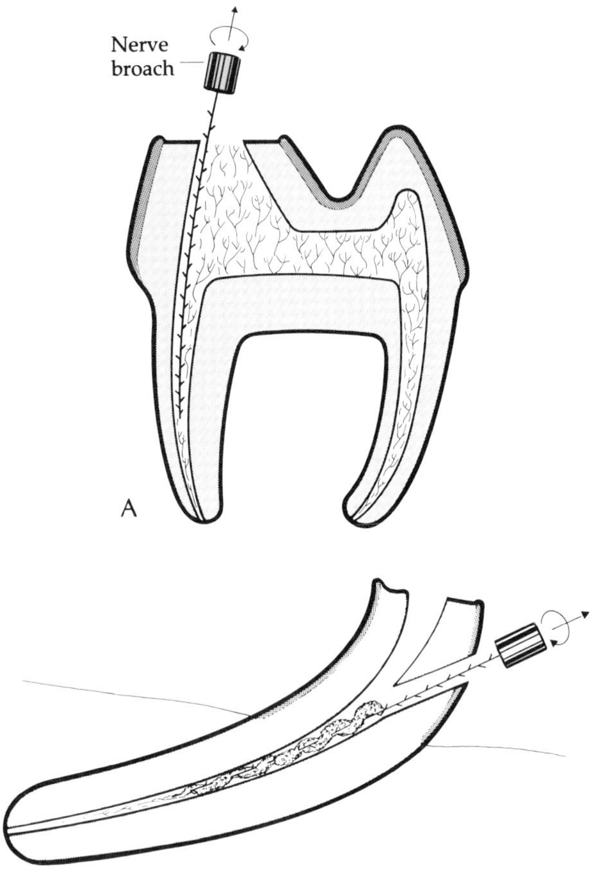

Fig. 6–8. *A*, Insertion of a nerve broach into the root canal; one carefully turns the broach by hand. *B*, Extraction of the pulp, threaded on the broach.

running the files into alveolar bone. In such a patient, the practitioner may have to perform an apicoectomy with retrograde filling to salvage the tooth.

The root canal is filled by means of a spiral root-canal filler (Lentulo-spiral). The creamy filling material is applied to the spiral, which is inserted into the root canal (Fig. 6–10); the spiral is slowly rotated while it is inserted. Careful to-and-fro motions strip off the filling material into the root canal. The rotating spiral is pressed against the root canal wall and is pulled out slowly in that position. The spiral should be cleaned immediately after use. If a spiral breaks during treatment, it may be left in the root canal.

To ensure that the filling material reaches the marginal areas of the pulp cavity, gutta-percha pins are inserted (Fig. 6–11). The root canal is completely filled when the filling material oozes out while the gutta-percha cone is inserted. One should examine the filling radiographically, to make sure it is free of air bubbles. The filling is then coated with pulp-protection cement. A permanent filling of amalgam or composite should be placed. In each case of tooth fracture, sharp enamel margins must be removed. If necessary, a crown restoration may be performed (Figs. 6–12 and 6–13).

If exposed pulp is not treated immediately, bacterial pulpitis may develop,

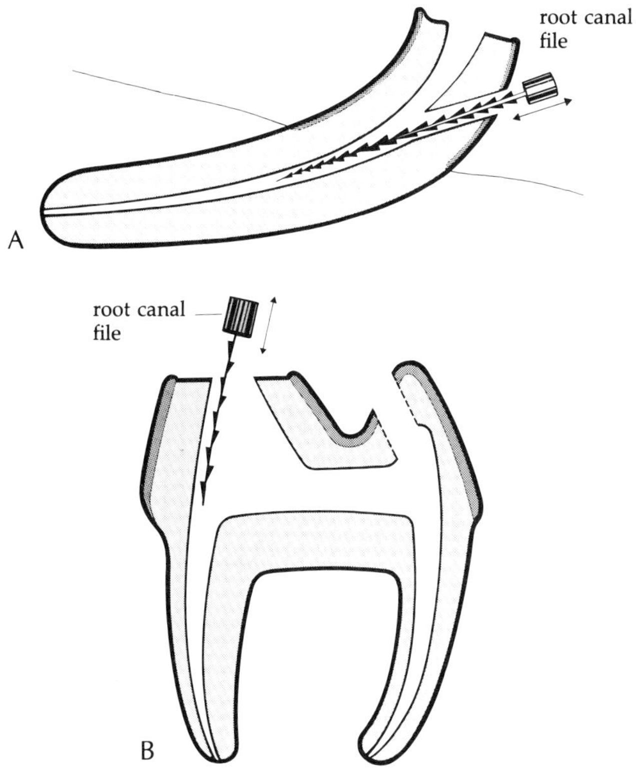

Fig. 6–9. *A*, Enlargement and planing of the root canal by means of root canal files. *B*, The same procedure as in *A*, but with a multirooted tooth.

eventually leading to necrosis. The infection may involve the periapical bone through the apical foramen, and may allow an acute periapical abscess to develop (Fig. 6–14). The risk is increased by preceding trauma to the periodontal membrane and periodontal ligament. Such an infection usually spreads, and acute alveolar periodontitis, osteomyelitis, and sepsis with severe general symptoms may develop as a consequence.

Loosened roots surrounded by pus are not tolerated by the body, which sheds the affected tooth. Such is especially true of the incisors and the double-rooted premolars in carnivores. The long roots of the canine teeth and, especially, the strong roots of the dog's canines are so firmly anchored in the jaw that these teeth become loose only after extended bone resorption. One or two of the roots of the canine tooth frequently remain sound and keep the tooth in its socket.

Chronic pulpitis and bacterial toxins in the pulp cavity initiate immunologic processes in the periapical tissue; in these processes, proliferous and destructive reactions take place simultaneously. Hyperemia, cellular infiltration, and edema raise the tissue pressure. The resorbed bone tissue is replaced by granulation tissue, which temporarily delays the spread of infection into the surrounding tissue. Thus, an apical granuloma develops; this lesion becomes visible as a periapical focus of absorption on a radiograph.

Often, no bacteria are found in the granuloma itself, at least not in the fiber-rich marginal areas. This aseptic condition can be disturbed by masticatory

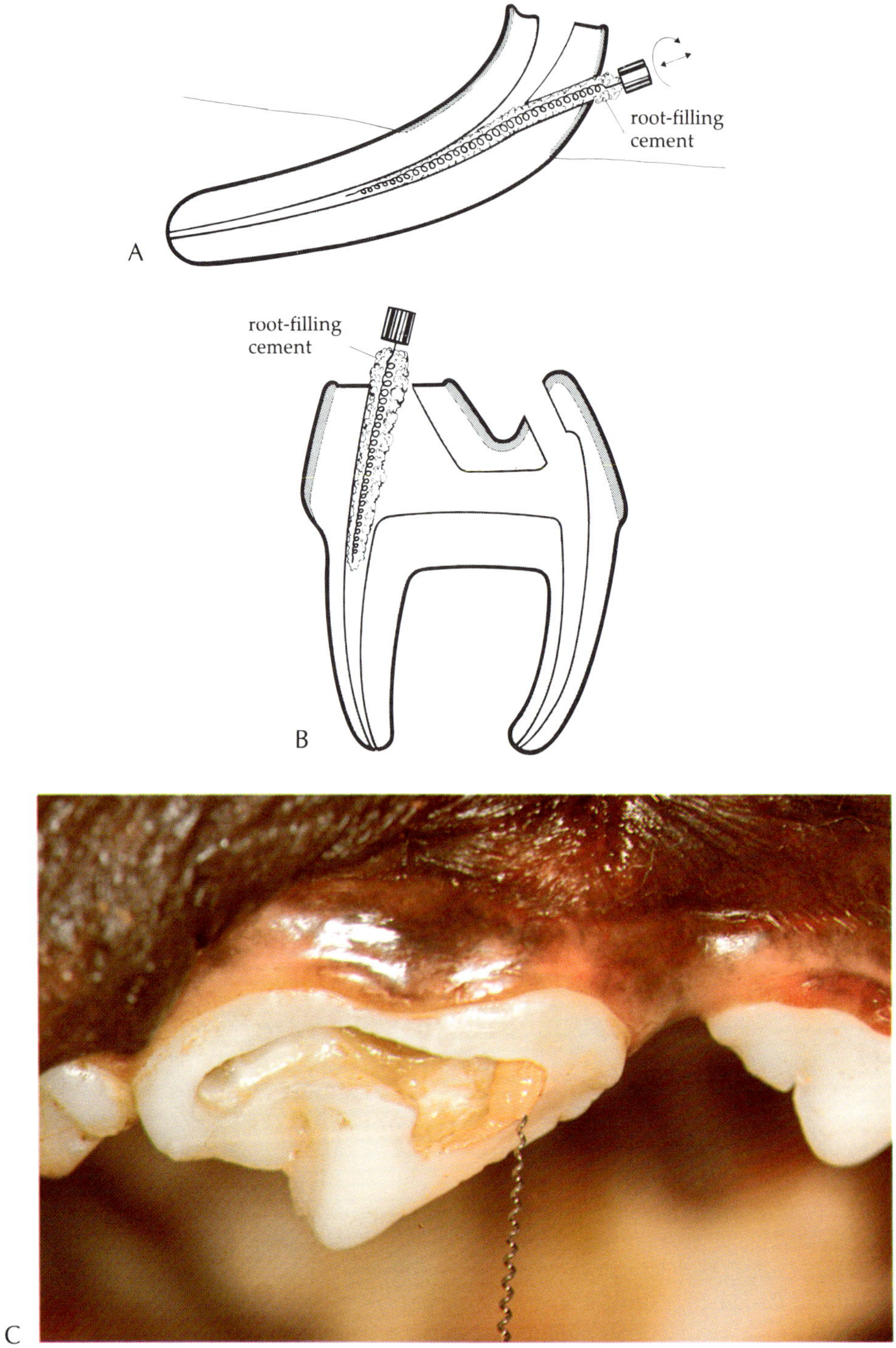

Fig. 6–10. *A,* Application of root-filling cement by means of an angle handpiece with slowly rotating spiral. *B,* The same procedure as in *A,* but with a multirooted tooth. *C,* Photograph of the root-filling process.

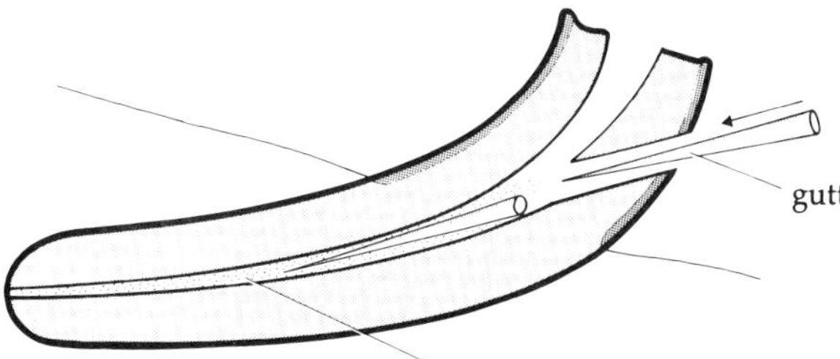

Fig. 6–11. Insertion of gutta-percha pins to ensure a complete filling.

pressure or by a weakened immune system. The granuloma then becomes septic and grows. The purulent infection may affect the periapical tissue and may cause a dental fistula or periodontitis to develop. The discharge of pus through the gingiva indicates that such a fistula has developed (Fig. 6–15).

The dental fistula, most often found in the dog, starts from P4 and erupts just below the eye through the skin as an external fistula (Fig. 6–16). Antibiotics have only a temporary effect, if any.

The granuloma may heal and may be replaced by bone tissue. This process can be instigated by treating the infected root, by mortal amputation or root canal filling, and in certain cases, by reducing the masticatory pressure by removing the crown or by feeding the patient soft food. Antibacterial agents, administered in high dosage parenterally or orally, are useful in this kind of treatment. Granulomas may also be treated permanently by root amputation.

If just one root of a multirooted tooth is fractured, it can be removed. The remaining tooth is treated endodontically, usually by vital amputation, without losing its masticatory function (the so-called "hemisection," Fig. 6–17).

TOOTH FRACTURE INVOLVING THE ALVEOLUS

Carnivores

Small tooth fragments should be removed. If the larger part of the root is uninjured, the exposed pulp can be treated, and a crown can be placed. Individual roots of multirooted teeth that are fractured or split deeply into the alveolus must be removed. The remaining tooth is treated endodontically.

Herbivores

The herbivore's posterior teeth nearly always fracture deeply into the alveolus longitudinally and must be removed. Loosened teeth with uninjured roots often

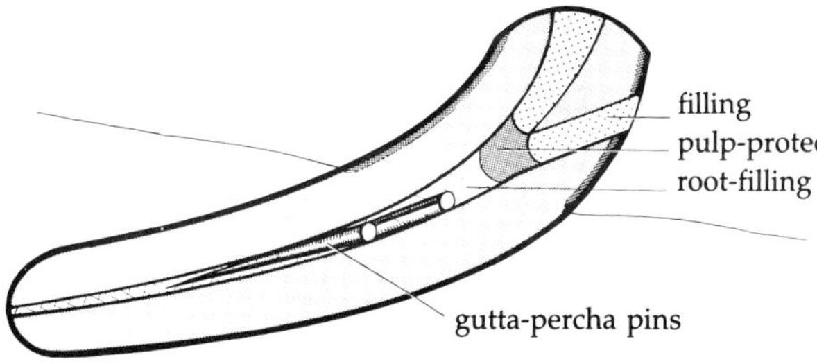

Fig. 6–12. Permanent filling; sharp edges of fracture have been rounded.

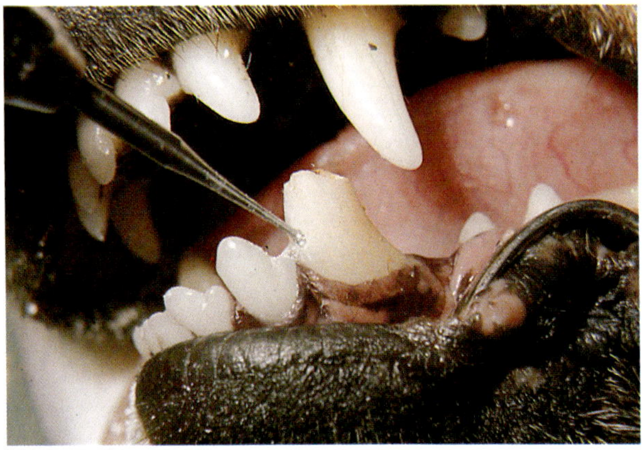

A

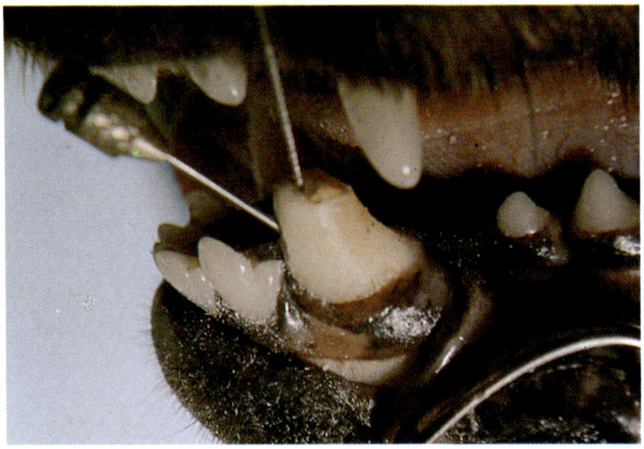

B

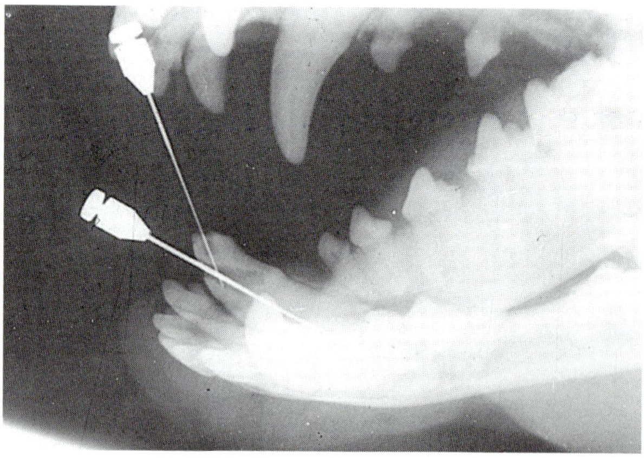

C

Fig. 6–13. *A* to *E*, Pulp extirpation and root-canal filling of a single-rooted tooth.

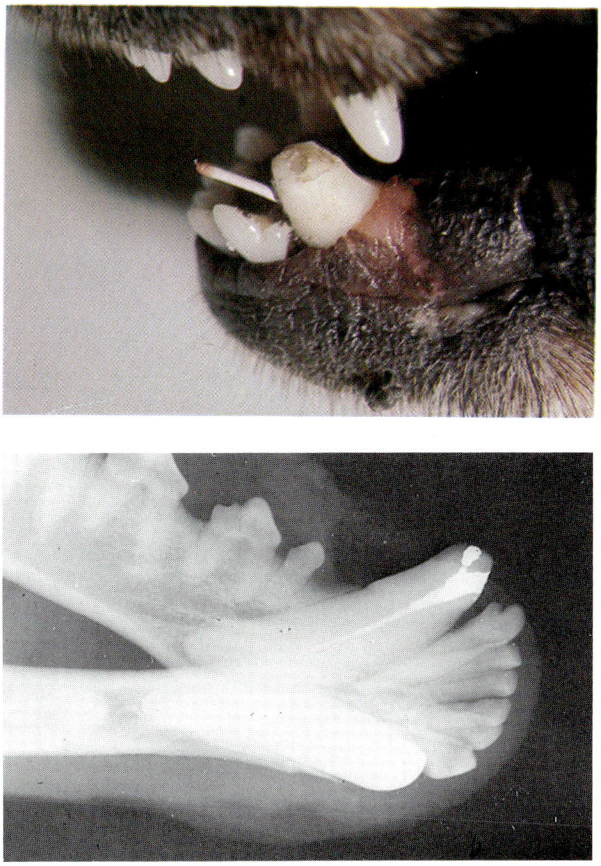

D

E

Fig. 6–13. ***Continued***

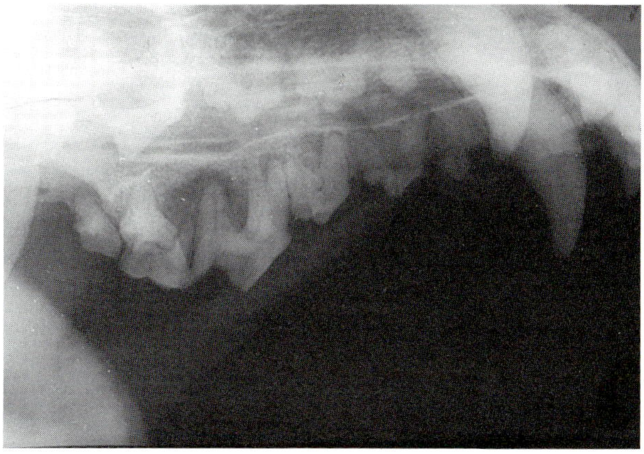

Fig. 6–14. Periapical resorption (granuloma) around the distal root of P4.

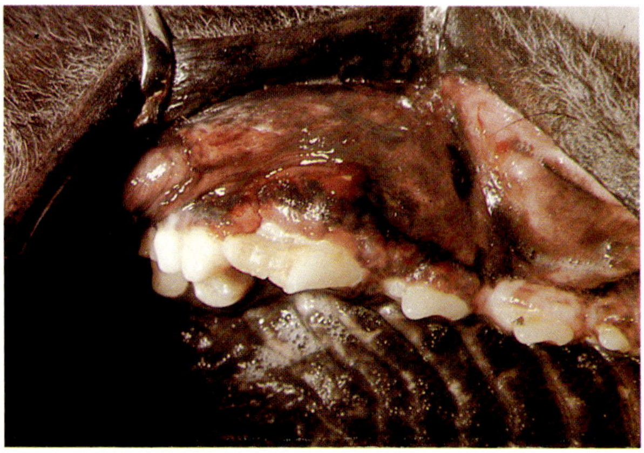

Fig. 6–15. Rare intraoral fistula from a previous fracture of P4. The fistula opening is about 1 cm above the gingival margin.

heal when they have been fixed in position and their occlusal surfaces have been ground down to avoid occlusal trauma against the antagonist teeth of the opposing jaw.

DENTAL FISTULA

Penetration of a periapical odontogenic abscess may cause a dental fistula. Infection of the periapical tissue follows pulpitis.

Dogs

The typical dental fistula penetrates the cheek below the eye and nearly always starts from a premolar (see Fig. 6–16); rarely does a dental fistula start from the root of a canine tooth.

Dental fistulas are usually caused by a slight fracture, although rarely they result from M1 caries or "periodontitis profunda," which is caused by the formation of subgingival tartar or impacted foreign bodies. The premolars are so firmly anchored in the jaw that a fistula develops before spontaneous shedding

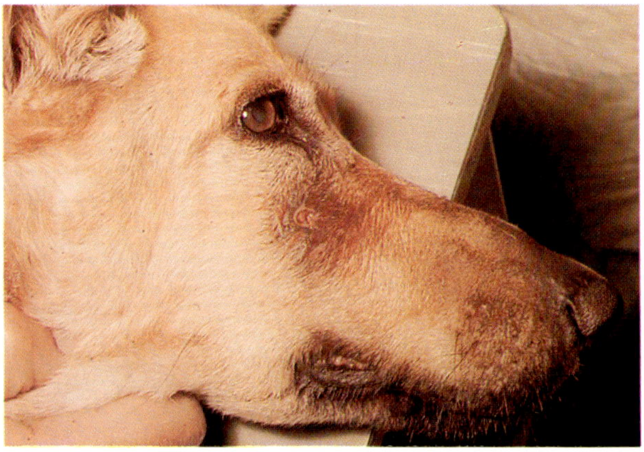

Fig. 6–16. Typical dentin fistula in dog, starting from P4.

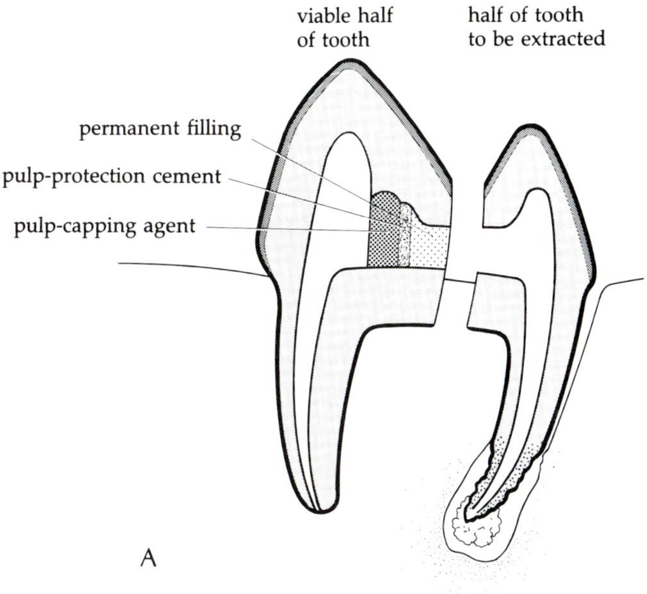

A

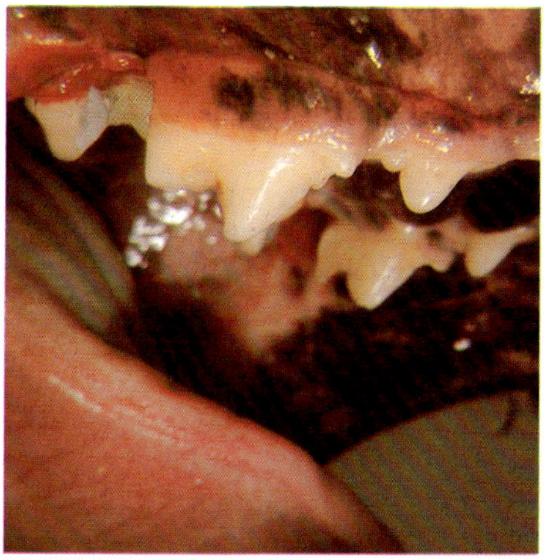

B

Fig. 6–17. *A*, Schematic view of hemisection of a multirooted tooth. *B*, Hemisection of the mesial root and crown of P4. The distal portion of the crown is filled with amalgam.

occurs. A fistula from P4 usually develops from only one of the three roots of this tooth; the other two roots maintain the partially vital tooth in its alveolus.

Symptoms

Before the fistula penetrates the skin, localized swelling becomes visible below the eye; in rare cases, half the face becomes edematous. The patient may suffer from lack of appetite and fever. The abscess finally penetrates the skin, leaving a fistulous lesion 1 to 2 mm in diameter. This opening, which continuously secretes small amounts of blood and pus, is surrounded by granular tissue and pigmented epithelium.

The premolar may have a yellowish brown soft point at the central apex, which is the opening of the pulp cavity. The tooth is usually firmly anchored and sometimes has a dirty, grayish yellow color. The radiograph shows a periapical resorption at one or two of the roots that may affect the roots of adjacent teeth.

Treatment

Heat treatment, soft food, and the administration of antibiotics may help an acute periapical granuloma to subside without developing into a fistula. A loosened tooth should be extracted; a fistula then heals spontaneously. An affected premolar that is firmly anchored and fully functional should be preserved by apicoectomy, especially in younger dogs.

Endodontic Therapy for Canine Teeth. In dogs and cats, endodontic therapy is indicated if pulp necrosis occurs. Pulp necrosis results whenever the pulp is exposed. Occasionally, this disorder follows hemorrhage of the pulp from severe trauma without direct fracture or exposure. Endodontic therapy is ineffective, however, when pulp necrosis occurs late in the course of periodontal disease. The pathophysiologic features of endodontic disease have been described. The sequence of events can be summarized as follows: pulp necrosis, apical granuloma formation, and acute apical abscess. The time required for this progression varies from months to years. An apical granuloma always forms after pulp necrosis, and this development necessitates therapeutic intervention.

Until recently, tooth extraction was the prevalent method of treating affected teeth, but currently available dental materials enable one to salvage teeth that might otherwise be lost. Although no two teeth are exactly the same and although the kinetics of function vary from the toy breeds to the large sighthounds, the principles of therapy are identical. The following technique has been used for several years with few postoperative failures.

All animals are maintained on halothane-nitrous oxide anesthesia. Intraoral radiographs of the involved tooth are taken, especially if the animal is less than a year old or if the surrounding bone exhibits a draining apical abscess. If the apex appears intact, an apicoectomy is not indicated. An apicoectomy is performed on the animal's canine teeth if radiographic evidence suggests apical root resorption or in a young animal with incomplete root development. Both these situations increase the likelihood of endodontic failure, thus necessitating the apicoectomy.

A routine root canal procedure on a canine tooth begins by palpating the buccal surface of the root structure. A straight line from the apex through the center of the tooth along its long axis is visualized. The exit point just above the gingival margin on the rostral portion of the tooth is the access hole that will be the entrance point for the root-canal files (Fig. 6–18*A*). A broken tooth crown may be so small that an access hole is not required, but it is important to maintain as straight a route as possible, to enable the files to reach the apex.

The access hole is made with a round carbide bur, in a position perpendicular to the tooth. Once through the enamel, the bur is redirected toward the apex until the bur enters the root canal. When the access hole is completed, reaming of the root canal begins. Fifty millimeter endodontic files are used, starting with a number 10 or 15 and finishing with up to a number 140. The first file is placed through the access hole and is pushed as far into the tooth as possible. Ideally,

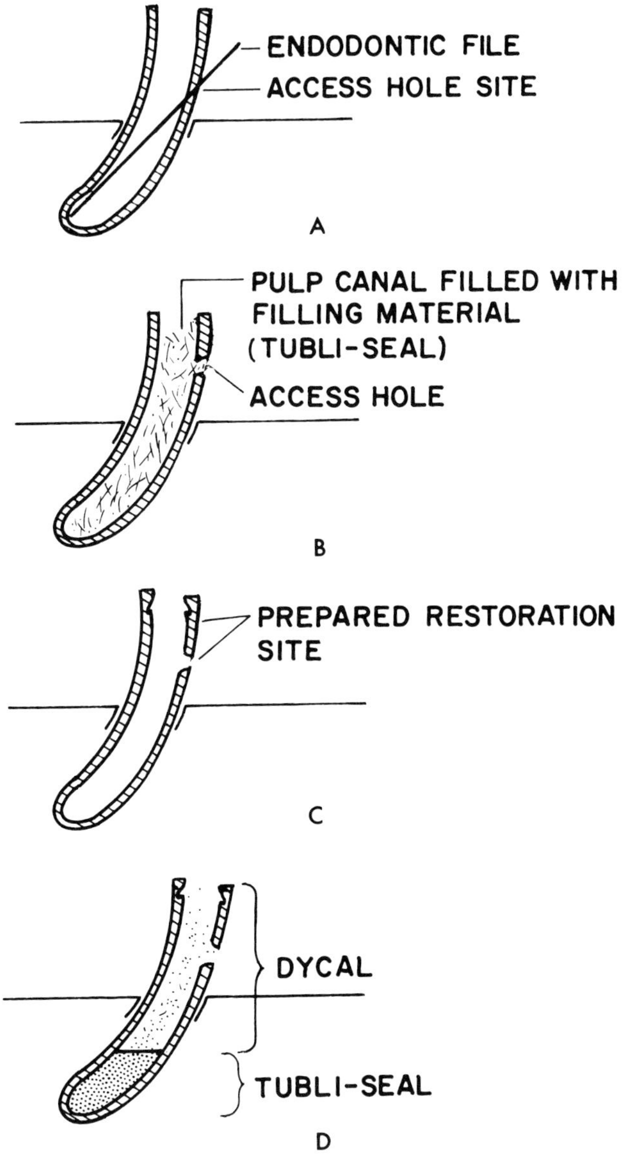

Fig. 6–18. See text for details.

the tooth should be radiographed to confirm that the tip of the file has reached the apex.

Once inside the tooth, the file is carefully rotated with a circular motion and then is withdrawn. Care is taken not to drive the file through the apex and also not to overtorque the file in the tooth. The tooth is periodically flushed, first with sodium hypochlorite, then with hydrogen peroxide, and finally with saline solution. Filing continues until the largest possible file, usually a number 80 to 120, removes only clean dentinal material. Next, the tooth root canal is dried with compressed air and paper points—long type-A points work best.

If apical hemorrhage cannot be controlled, the apex should be irrigated with lidocaine and 2% epinephrine by placing a 1.5 inch, 22-gauge needle through the access hole. If this procedure does not control apical hemorrhage in a few minutes, an apicoectomy should be performed. Once the root canal is dried, canal sealer is placed in the root canal. One requires approximately 0.5 to 1.0 ml mixture to fill the average tooth. The animal's head is placed so the apex is down. The needle is inserted into the access hole as far as it will go, and the tubuli sealing agent (Tubli-Seal) is pressed into the tooth until it is full (Fig. 6–18*B*). The needle is slowly backed out of the hole; one must ensure that the tubuli sealant fills the tooth while the needle is removed. Next, the mixture is allowed to air dry for approximately 5 minutes; any excess is removed. An inverted cone bur is used to carve a seat for the amalgam fillings in both the access hole and the fracture site in the crown (Fig. 6–18C). Amalgam fillings are placed, and the animal is allowed to awaken. The owners are instructed to feed only a light meal that night and to resume normal activity the next day.

A variation of this technique is recommended for young dogs with huge root canals and thin dentinal walls. This variation can also be used if amalgam is not available and if the practitioner is using a composite-resin restorative material. This composite is not compatible with the tubuli sealing agent. The sealant is placed on the apex as described, but only enough to fill the apex (Fig. 6–18*D*). The remaining space is filled with Dycal caulk to strengthen the crown and also to act as an interface against the composite. The working time with this type of caulk is short. A 1.5-inch, 20-gauge needle is needed to insert the material; the practitioner must move quickly. The caulk is placed over the tubuli sealing agent at the apex, and the remainder of the root canal and crown are filled. An inverted cone bur is used to carve a seat for the amalgam fillings in both the access hole and the fracture site in the crown. An amalgam or composite restoration is placed, and the animal is allowed to awaken.

For teeth requiring an apicoectomy, the length of the root canal is measured by placing a file in the root canal and radiographing the tooth. The file is marked at the access hole and then is removed from the tooth and is placed over the tooth on the buccal surface, for maxillary teeth, and on the ventral surface, for mandibular teeth. Next, the gingiva (or skin) is infiltrated with lidocaine and 2% epinephrine over the apex to control hemorrhage. For mandibular teeth, sterile technique is used; a skin incision allows access to the apex site on the ventral surface of the mandible. For maxillary teeth, an incision through the gingiva accomplishes the same end. A No. 5 sterile carbide bur is used to remove bone over the apex. The measured root-canal file is used as a reference to pin point the apex. Once the root canal is opened, the standard root-canal technique is completed. A retrograde amalgam carrier is used to place the filling at the apex. Care must be taken to seal the apex and to keep the operative field dry. Once the filling has been placed, the gingiva or skin is closed, and the procedure is completed on the crown. Antibiotics are desirable for 10 days postoperatively to expedite healing.

Apicoectomy (Fig. 6–19). Before removing the root apex, the pulp cavity must be opened, and the residual pulp must be extirpated. Treatment and disinfection of root canals have been described earlier. A root-canal instrument is inserted into the root in question (Fig. 6–19*A*), and it is pulled out again after one marks the depth of insertion. Finally, the position of the root apex is marked

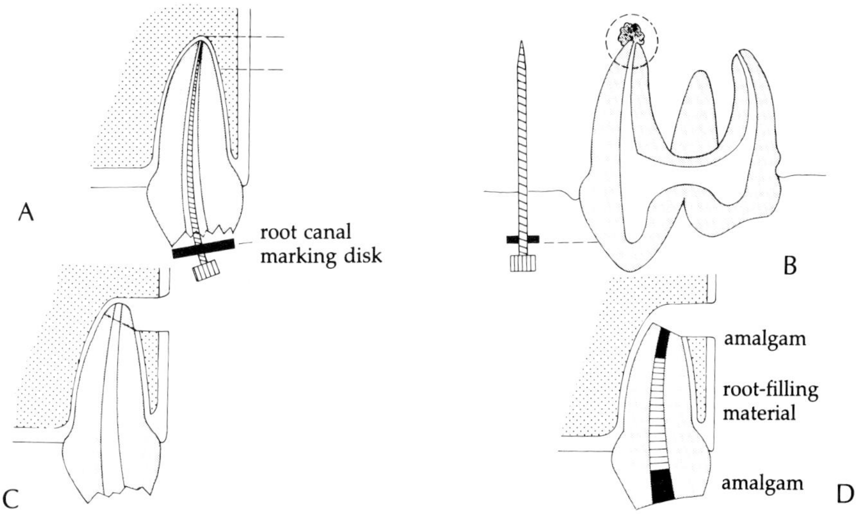

Fig. 6–19. Schematic view of apicoectomy. *A*, Insertion of a root-canal instrument and marking of the depth of insertion. *B*, Finding the position of the root apex outside on the mucosa with a root-canal instrument. *C*, Preparation of the alveolar wall and exposure of the root. *D*, Oblique dissection of the root apex and filling of the exposed root canal.

on the mucosa (Fig. 6–19*B*). The buccal as well as the labial mucosa are then incised (Fig. 6–20). The incision is made parallel to the root.

The periosteum is incised to expose a large area of the bone surface. Hemorrhage is controlled with a local infiltration of lidocaine or epinephrine. In the maxilla, near the sectorial tooth, attention should be paid to the nerves and vessels of the infraorbital foramen. The outer alveolar wall is trephined in a circular way with a round bur or a small trephine. When the bone disk has been removed, the root apex becomes visible (Figs. 6–19*C*, 6–21, and 6–22). It is obliquely dissected with a fissure bur in a high-speed handpiece (see Fig. 6–19*D*)

The apical root canal is enlarged to hold the amalgam filling. The root canal should be checked by inserting an explorer from the crown. The explorer point should be visible at the removed area of the root apex.

After repeated disinfection, hemostasis, and drying, the root apex should be filled with amalgam. The root canal should be filled as described earlier. Care should be taken not to insert the filling material too deeply and thereby to push out the apically applied amalgam filling. The crown cavity should then be permanently filled with amalgam or composite (Fig. 6–23).

Horses

The typical dental fistula in the horse occurs in the mandible. It mainly affects horses between the ages of 2 and 5 years and usually starts from P4, P3, and M1 (Fig. 6–24).

Causes include temporary tooth retention, unequal rate of growth of permanent premolars, loosening and infection of the periodontium caused by change of teeth, unusual masticatory or growth pressure of the dental sac, hematogenous infection of the affected periapical tissue, and caries or tooth fracture after cemental hypoplasia.

Signs of a dental fistula in horses include hard swelling of the mandible,

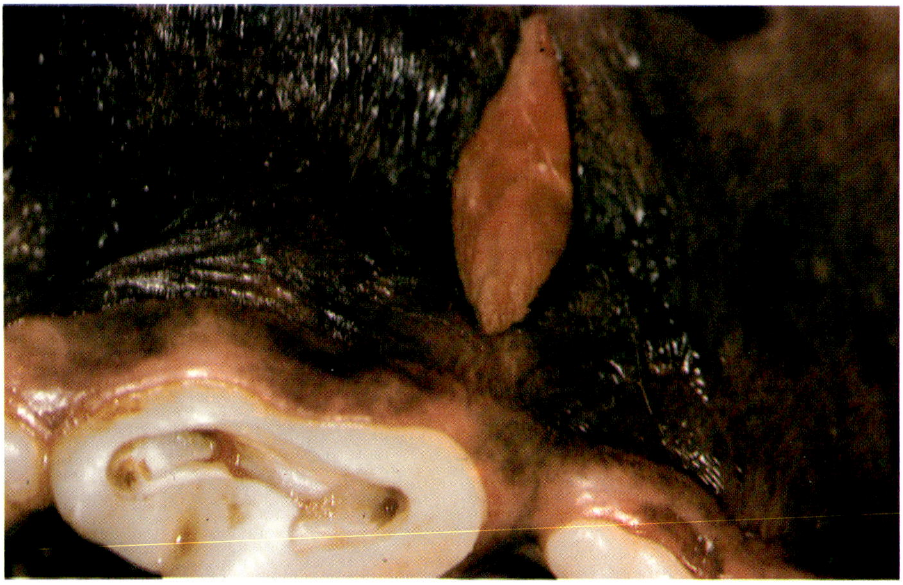

Fig. 6–20. Apicoectomy in a dog; vertical incision over the mesial root apex.

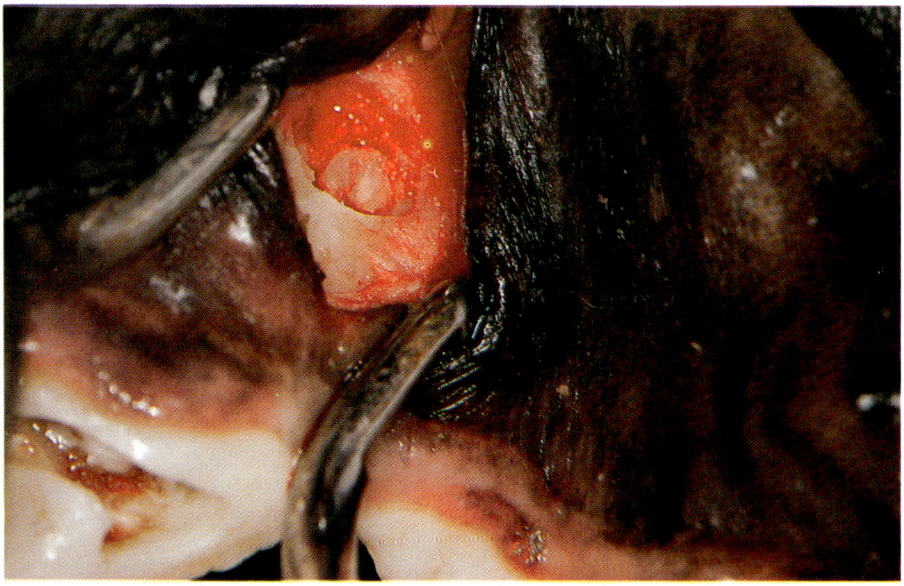

Fig. 6–21. The root apex is visible after trephining the jaw bone.

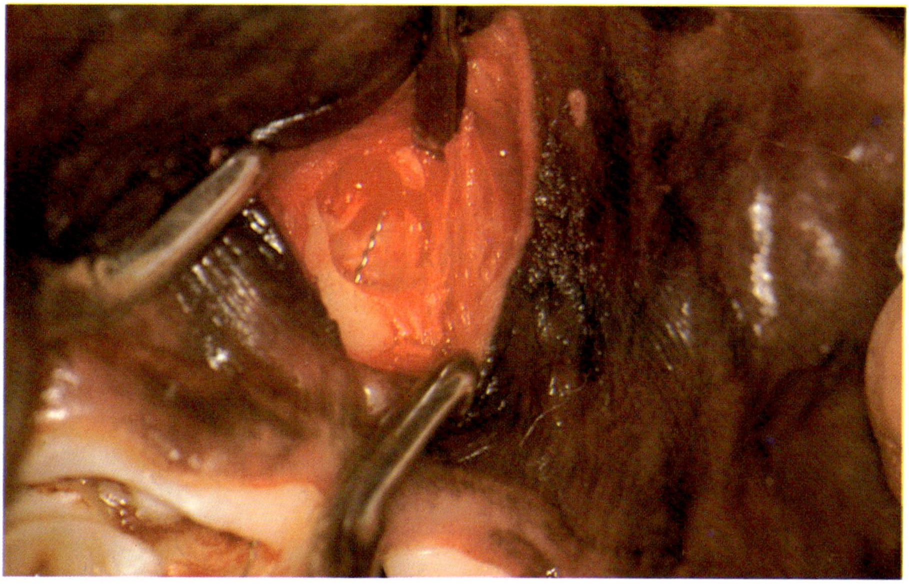

Fig. 6–22. The crownward-inserted explorer appears at the apical root opening.

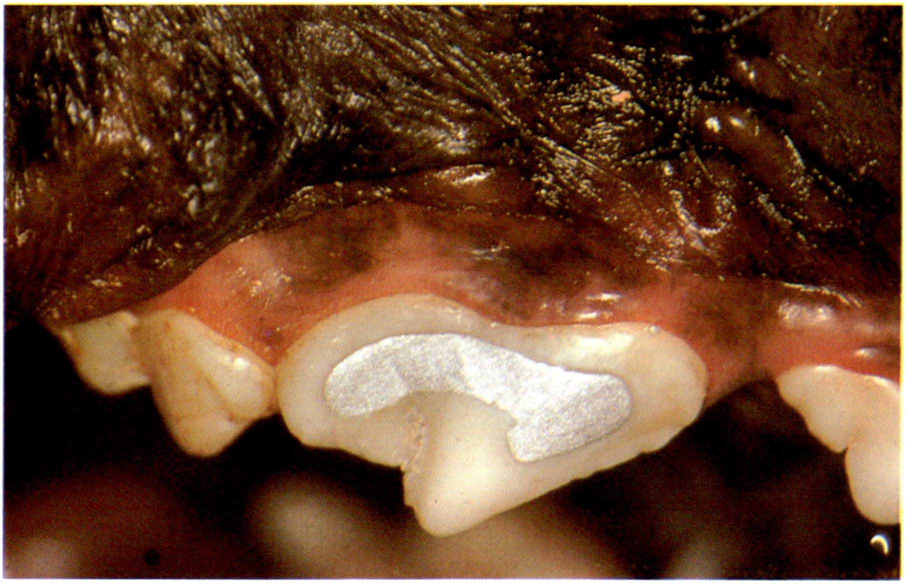

Fig. 6–23. Permanent filling with amalgam.

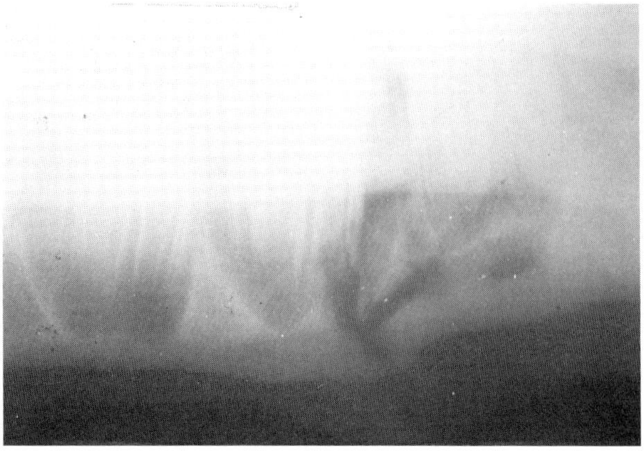

Fig. 6–24. Dental fistula in a horse. The fistula canal and a sequestrum are visible in the radiograph. The adjacent teeth show a limited dental sac.

penetration of an abscess, a short phase of an edematous cellulitis, and finally, formation of a permanent fistula. When using a metal explorer, the dull, crunching sound of touching bone can often be distinguished from the clear, hard sound of touching a tooth. In the maxilla, pus penetrates the maxillary sinus. Consequently, a foul-smelling, one-sided nasal discharge or a swelling of the maxilla is caused (empyema).

Indistinctly contoured bone resorptions, possibly with an osseous canal to the fistula opening, can be seen against the jaw in radiographs. On the other hand, the enlarged sterile dental sacs in colts and foals are distinctly limited and have a hooded appearance around the root apex.

Treatment

Apicoectomy is the preferred treatment for a dental fistula (Fig. 6–25). The fistula should be dissected. Large-scale lateral trephining, with a trephine or a chisel, of the jaw bone above the root apex and oblique dissection of the root apex with an air drill should be performed (Fig. 6–25*A*). The narrow root canal should be widened, and any residual pulp should be extirpated (Fig. 6–25*B*). Then, the pulp cavity should be cleaned, disinfected, and filled with antibacterial root-filling paste, such as Formocresol. Finally, the cavity should be filled with amalgam (Fig. 6–25C). The use of a suction apparatus is recommended for maintaining a dry operation site. After filling, the periapical tissue must be curetted and rinsed, and antibiotics should be prescribed. Drainage, wound closure, and healing may be enhanced by a slight shortening of the crown of the affected tooth.

TOOTH EXTRACTION

The tooth is attached to the bony alveolus by the strong Sharpey's fibers and the elastic but firm gingiva. The firm anchorage in the connective tissue can be deteriorated by inflammation. A further loosening of the tooth can occur in response to a periapical granuloma or by bone recession of the alveolar margin due to periodontitis. Teeth in older animals, which have shortened roots, as well as teeth with a changed periodontium, are much easier to extract than teeth in younger animals or teeth with several long and curved roots. Before extraction is performed, the gingiva must be separated as far as the alveolar margin with a periosteal elevator, a gouge, or Bein's elevator, lest the gingiva be injured under strong tension.

If the alveolus can be easily reached, as in the dentition of small animals and the incisors of large animals, one should attempt to insert Bein's elevator with to-and-fro motions at several different points between the alveolar margin and the root. Roots loosened in this way are much easier to extract. The blades of the forceps should be slightly curved and serrated, but they should not have a sharp point, such as forceps in human dentistry, because such a point may fracture the tooth. The forceps are placed near the alveolar margin and, according to the looseness of the tooth, are moved to obtain a shorter hold to facilitate removal.

Dogs

To extract a dog's incisor, one should rotate the forceps slowly along the longitudinal axis of the root.

To extract a canine tooth, the lateral alveolar wall along the strong root is exposed by incision of the gingiva and is removed with a gouge. Burs and handpieces are also suited for this purpose. Only loose canine teeth can be extracted with forceps (rotating motions) or with Bein's elevator.

Two-rooted premolars are extracted by loosening with light to-and-fro motions. Isolating each root by using a diamond cutting wheel or a carbide bur facilitates extraction.

Loosened three-rooted premolars and molars can be further loosened by careful to-and-fro motions; at least one root should be affected by a granuloma or by resorption of the alveolar wall. When the highest degree of looseness has been reached, squelching sounds can be heard as blood and air are sucked into the alveolus.

A broken root is loosened by means of Bein's elevator and is extracted. Such a root can also be gripped and pulled out with a pair of slender root forceps. Rarely must the alveolar wall be trephined. The crowns of firmly anchored three-rooted teeth are separated by a handpiece, so each root can be removed independently.

Cats

The cat's thin incisor roots often break during extraction.

As in dogs, the thin roots of the cat's canines and premolars must be loosened carefully, especially in the mandible, to avoid fracturing the jaw. Roots or root fragments that remain in the jaw are best trimmed with a rose-head bur.

The crowns of the firmly anchored three-rooted posterior teeth are removed with a handpiece, and the roots are trimmed from the alveolus. Slender gouges or Bein's elevators can also be used to loosen the roots of teeth.

Horses

To avoid injuring the patient, the assistant, or the practitioner, tooth extraction should be performed with the patient's head firmly fixed using an appropriate fixation apparatus. The operation is facilitated if the horse is lying down.

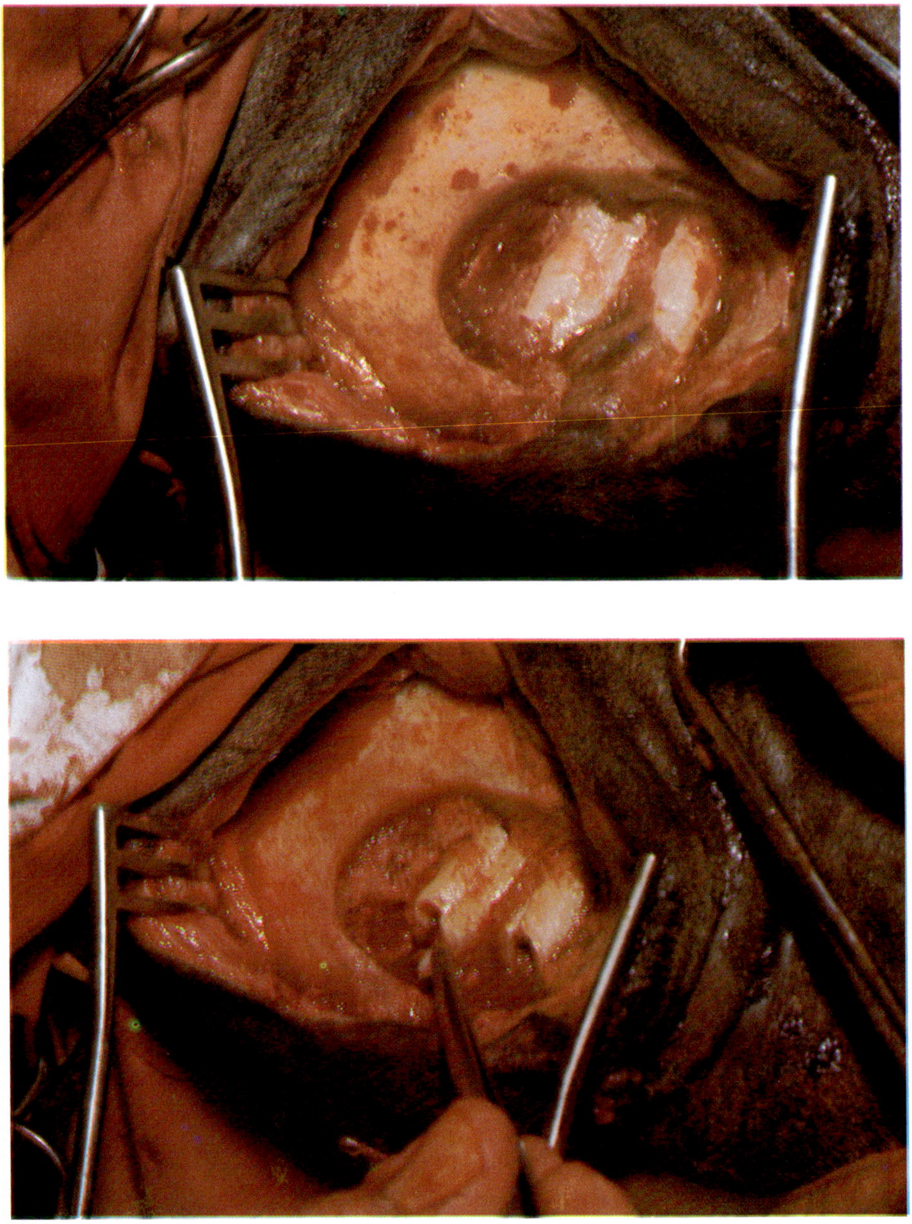

A

B

Fig. 6–25. Apicoectomy in a horse. *A,* The roots in the mandible of a horse become visible after trephining the outer alveolar wall. *B,* Extirpation of the residual pulp.

C 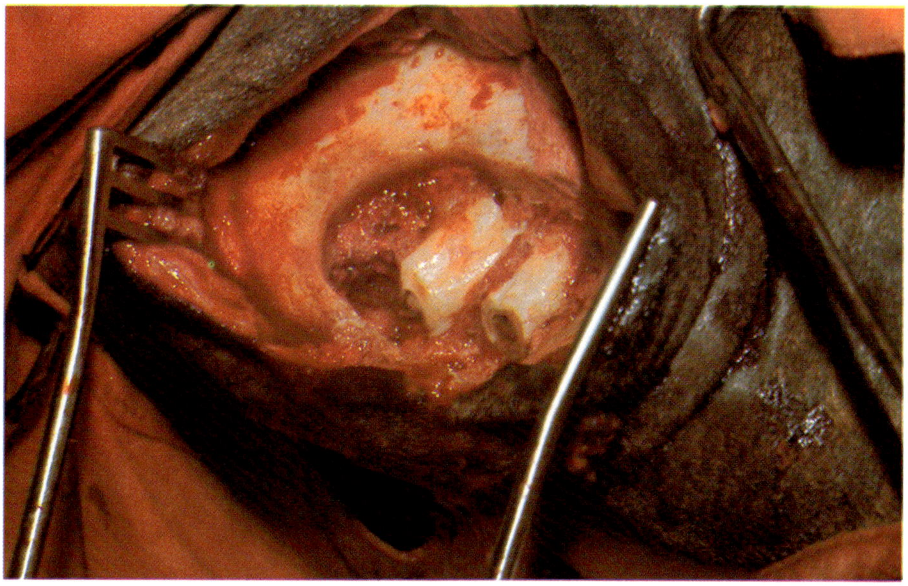

Fig. 6–25. *Continued* *C*, Pulp cavity filled with amalgam.

The incisors are extracted by enlarging the alveolus with a chisel and by gently rotating the forceps along the longitudinal axis of the tooth.

Locating a diseased posterior tooth is facilitated by radiography.

The forceps should have long flexible handles and flat blades. The blades of the forceps should firmly grip the tooth to be extracted, and the handles should be bound together to maintain the grip. Rotational motions along the longitudinal axis of the tooth are then performed. A tooth loosened in this way can often be pulled out by hand; if such is not possible, a piece of wood should be placed under the hinge of the forceps, for leverage.

It is often difficult to remove the long aboral posterior teeth because of lack of space. They cannot be pulled out whole because they are blocked by the opposing teeth. The crown of the tooth must therefore be cut with shears once or twice, to shorten the tooth until it can be removed.

The mandibular teeth and the maxillary posterior teeth, which are accessible through the maxillary sinuses, can be driven from their sockets and expelled into the oral cavity with a metal punch and a mallet after trephining and exposing the root. Care should be taken to localize the tooth to be expelled; tooth fragments are removed with a sharp curette or with splinter forceps. Expulsion is particularly indicated for fractured teeth or for those with broken crowns.

The expulsion of aboral posterior teeth is nearly impossible because of the masseter muscle that lies between them and the cheek and makes it difficult to gain access to the tooth to be expelled; on the other hand, it is rarely necessary to extract these teeth. When a tooth has been expelled, an opening leads from the oral cavity, through the alveolus, and into the bone or maxillary sinus, into which soft food might be pressed. This opening should therefore be packed with antiseptic gauze or dental wax until it fills with granulation tissue in about 10 days. A strong silk thread is tied to an elastic piece of rubber or gauze packing. The rubber or gauze should be large enough not to be pulled into the maxillary sinus through the alveolus; the thread should be passed through the opening to the outside through the incision made to perform the expulsion. There it should be fixed by means of an elastic rubber hose about as thick as a finger; pulling the thread through the hose prevents it from slipping. In about 2 weeks, the thread is cut, and the gauze packing is removed through the oral cavity or is spat out by the patient. In horses younger than 8 years old, none of the posterior teeth should be extracted unless they are loose or fractured; until horses are at least 8 years old, antagonist teeth will grow into the interdental spaces caused by extractions. This process is due to active elongation and lack of abrasion; unapposed teeth eventually assume the shape of a chisel.

JAW AND ALVEOLAR FRACTURES

Jaw fractures are nearly always open fractures because the periosteum and the firmly attached gingiva have little elasticity and tear above the site of fracture. Such is particularly true for alveolar fractures.

Various surgical techniques are available, such as the application of external splinting, dynamic-compression plates, and intramedullary pins. Care should be taken to preserve the roots of adjacent teeth that are not yet fully developed. Fixation with a temporary composite bridge that includes the incisors and canines is also recommended.

Intraoral treatment is based on the tendency of the gingiva and the periodontium to heal, provided the patient's condition stabilizes quickly, before fundamental infectious and necrotic changes occur.

Loss and Dislocation of Single Teeth or Groups of Teeth

The prognosis is encouraging if the jaw itself is not broken. This type of injury occurs in horses when they are kicked by other horses or when they fall. In dogs, it occurs as a result of bites, fights, beatings, and other sorts of accidents (Fig. 6–26*A*).

Treatment

Foreign bodies, such as hairs, crushed bone fragments, and blood clots should be removed from the area of fracture, the alveolar wall, and the root. Wounds that are not fresh should be scraped clean and washed with an antibiotic solution. The gingiva should be tightly sutured. Antibiotics should be administered parenterally.

Fixation. Wire loops are laid around the dislocated teeth and the firmly anchored adjacent teeth, or through boreholes in the jaw bone. If necessary, the loops can be fixed with additional acrylate or composite (Fig. 6–26*B*).

A successful technique in horses and dogs consists of grinding a groove into the dislocated teeth; a wire splint is then cemented into this groove. In dogs, the groove is ground into the tooth wall. In horses, the groove is ground into the occlusal surfaces of the incisors. By carefully grinding the occlusal surface, one ensures that the repositioned teeth in herbivores are temporarily free of any masticatory pressure (Fig. 6–27).

Fractures of the Symphysis

Fracture of the symphysis occurs almost exclusively in carnivores. A figure-eight wire loop is laid around the canine teeth. In certain cases, the stabilizing

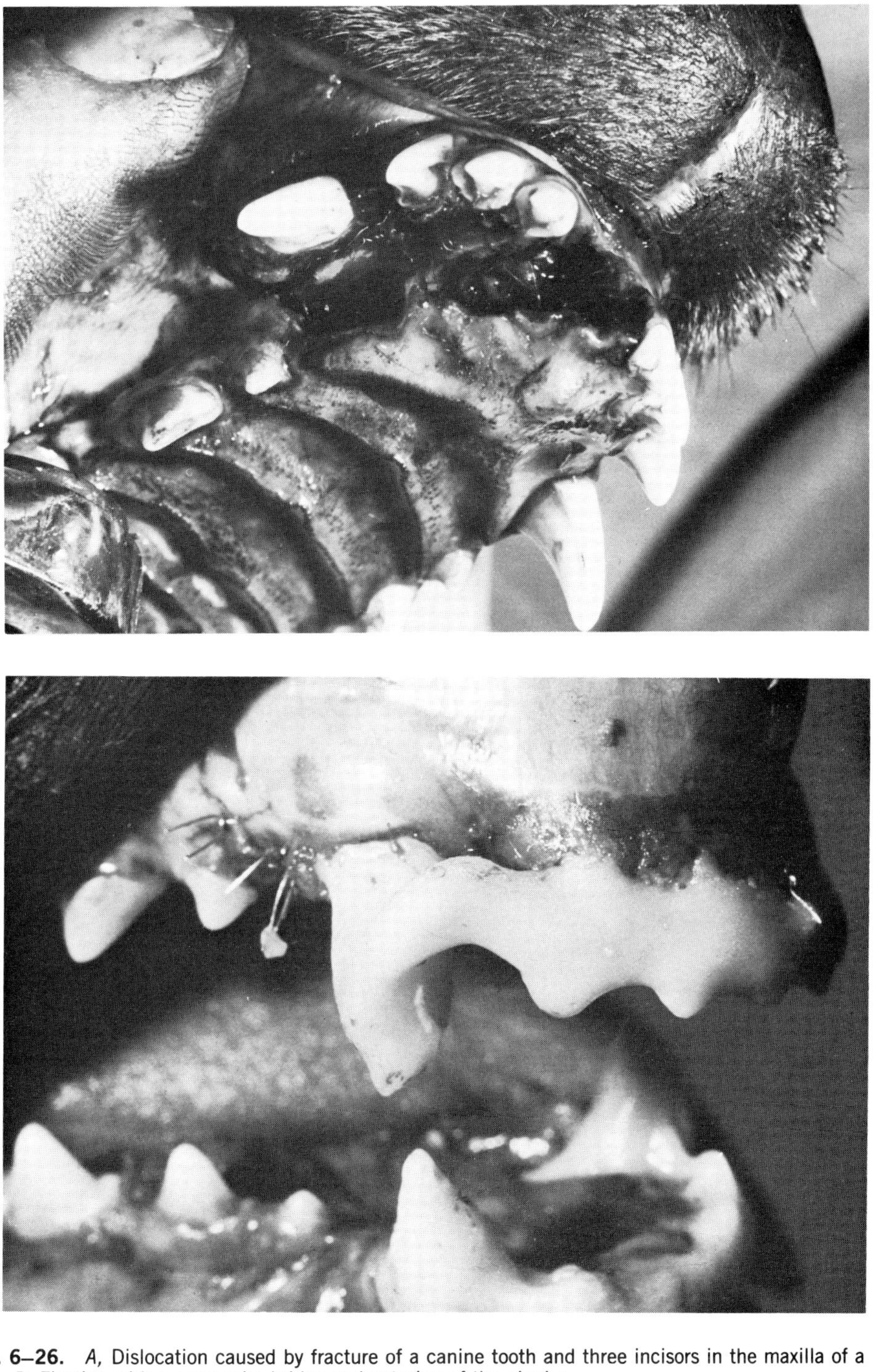

A

B

Fig. 6–26. *A*, Dislocation caused by fracture of a canine tooth and three incisors in the maxilla of a dog. *B*, Fixation with a composite bridge and suturing of the gingiva.

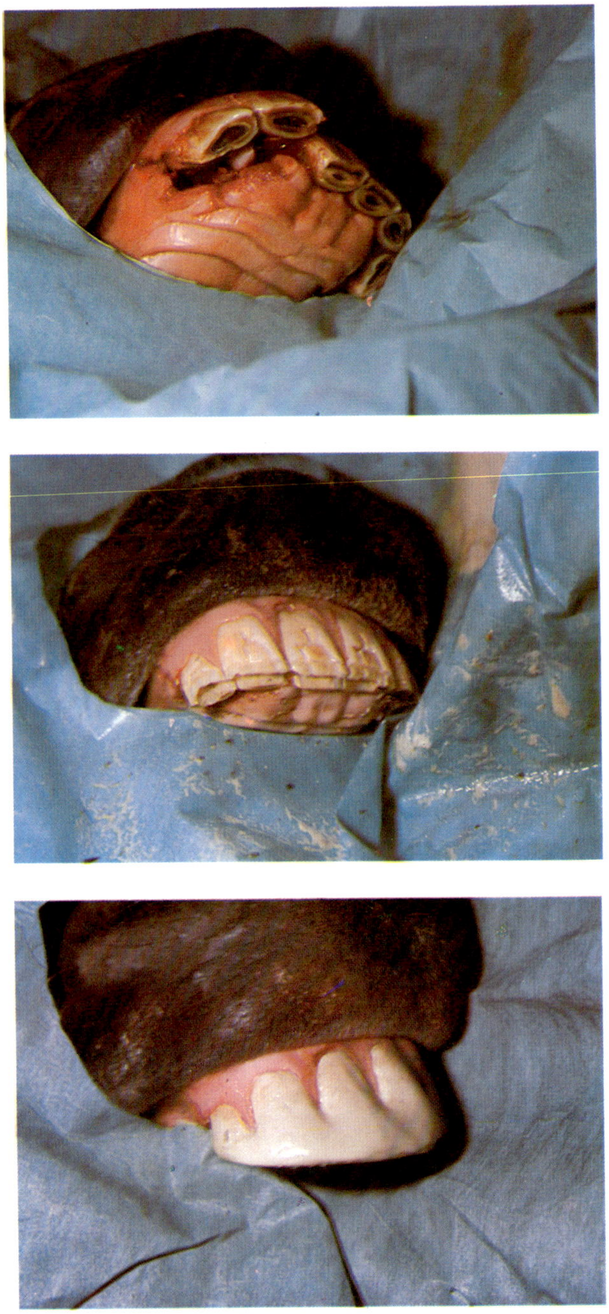

A

B

C

Fig. 6–27. *A,* Dislocation of I2 and I3 in a horse. *B,* Milling a snow-tire tread profile into the labial surfaces of the incisors; deepening and connecting the infundibuli with a groove. An alternate treatment is the labial application of Thread-Mate System pins to retain the composite bridge. *C,* Fixation with the composite bridge.

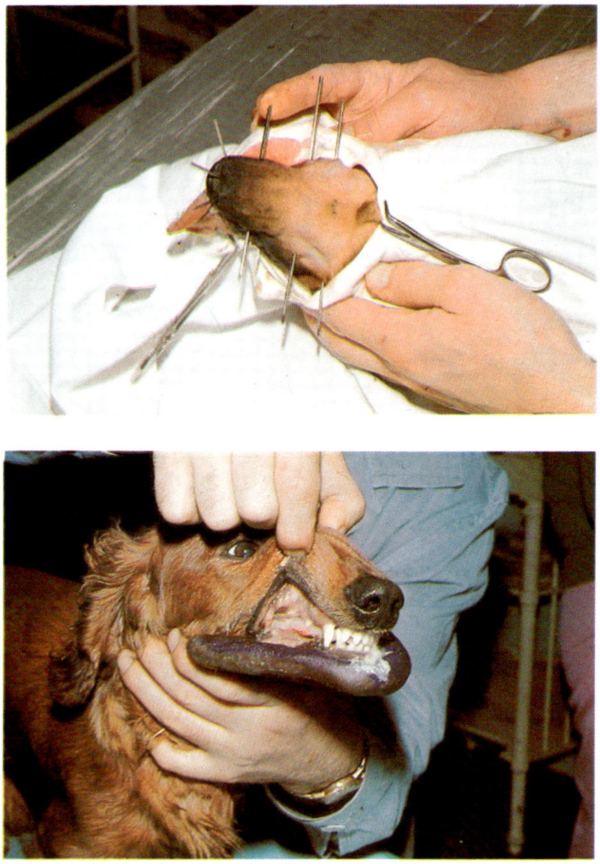

A

B

Fig. 6–28. *A*, Bilateral mandible fracture: splint fixation. The posterior splints penetrate both mandibles; the anterior, radially positioned splints are inserted into the bone near the incisors. *B*, Stabilizing the splints with acrylate.

effect is even better if the loop is laid submucously around the jaw bones. Displacement of either half of the jaw can be prevented by a transversely bored pin. Care should be taken to preserve the roots of the canine teeth.

Splinting

For splinting fractures near the posterior teeth and of the mandibular articular process, the canines can be used in carnivores. The mouth of long-nosed breeds of dogs is tied with a band for 2 to 3 weeks. The maxilla and the mandible in cats can be sutured subgingivally with steel wire; however, the danger of infection is great. High doses of antibiotics and frequent examinations are essential.

Tying the mouth with bands that are glued to the cast or are applied with adhesive tape is recommended for quiet animals only.

Recommended Treatment for Cats

One TMS pin is inserted into each of the maxillary and mandibular canine teeth, to reposition the jaws; fixation is achieved by a composite bridge between the pins. The animal is fed a liquid-pulpy food through the cheek opening. The bridge can be removed in 2 to 3 weeks.

Fractures of the Mandible

Fractures of the mandible occur in the diastema in horses and in the molar region in carnivores. These fractures can be fixed with wire loops alone or with additional extraoral apparatus. The effectiveness of the tension-wire technique is enhanced by muscle pull. The wire is laid through a bore hole close above the bony alveolar margin between the teeth, and then it is tightened. External splinting with wire loops and acrylate bridging has proved successful in treating mandibular fractures of dogs (Fig. 6–28).

Fractures of the Maxilla

Other than the repositioning of individual teeth or groups of teeth and suturing of the mucosa, maxillary fractures do not call for any special stabilizing techniques because they are fixed by the physiologically elastic elements of the face.

Bibliography: 1, 3, 5, 6, 7, 8, 9, 10, 11, 17, 18, 20, 21, 23, 26, 29, 37, 39, 40, 42, 43, 44, 46, 47, 52, 53, 54, 58, 59, 61

7

Crown and Tooth Restoration

RESTORATION WITH THE ACID-ETCH TECHNIQUE

Indications

Reconstruction of a fractured tooth crown with the acid-etch technique is indicated if enough enamel is present. If more than half a crown has been lost, restoration with an adhesive technique without additional anchorage cannot be recommended.

The advantage of adhesive restoration is that the pulp is protected because the dental tubules exposed by the tooth fracture are sealed, and bacterial and thermal irritations are thereby prevented from reaching the pulp through the composite. Because of satisfactory aesthetic appearance, this kind of restoration is recommended to owners of exhibition animals.

Technique

If the pulp is exposed, endodontic treatment must be performed first. Then, the enamel area close to the fracture must be cleaned with pumice on a rotating brush or a polishing rubber cup (Fig. 7–1). In this process, the superficial necrotic layers are removed, to assist the adhesion of the composite. If the pulp is not exposed, but lies just below the fractured surface and shines, rose colored, through the dentin, one must either perform indirect pulp capping with calcium hydroxide or seal the dental tubules with cavity liners, to avoid later irritation of the pulp by the composite. If the pulp is far below the fracture, as in an apical fracture of a canine tooth, indirect capping need not be performed. Before proceeding with the etching, the tooth should be isolated with a thin rubber dam to keep moisture and saliva away from the area to be etched.

The enamel surface surrounding the fracture must be etched with phosphoric acid (Figs. 7–2 and 7–3). Different etching preparations, such as gels and solutions, are available from various manufacturers. The manufacturer's instructions should be followed strictly. After the prescribed etching time, usually 60 seconds, the etching liquid is sprayed off with an oil-free water spray. Is is not advisable to use the dental turbine's spray apparatus because it may contain tiny traces of oil. If no dental spray equipment is at hand, a clean plastic dis-

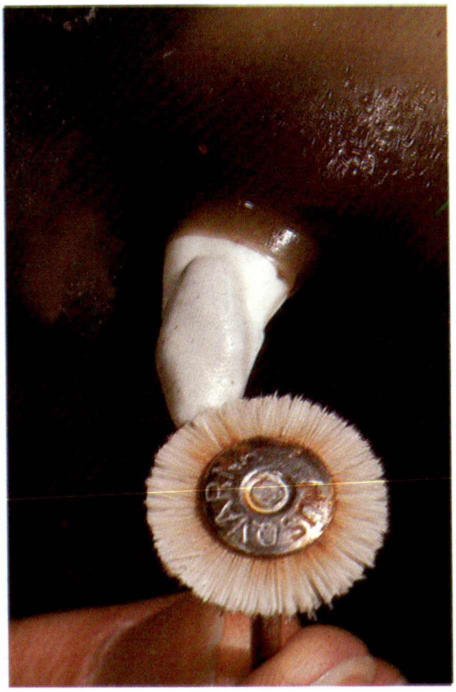

Fig. 7–1. Cleaning with a rotating brush and pumice; the tooth is isolated by a rubber dam.

posable syringe with a thin needle should be used. An oil-free spray is absolutely necessary because the least trace of oil affects the adhesion of the composite and the durability of the restoration. With this technique, the enamel prisms are etched to a depth of 10 μm. These indentations enlarge the enamel surface immensely and are necessary for the micromechanical anchorage of the composite that flows into and fills these pores. The loss of enamel thickness is negligible, about 1%. Accidentally etched teeth are remineralized within 48 hours by salivary mineral salts.

After thoroughly spraying off the etching liquid, the enamel is dried with an air blower that contains no oil. Provided etching is performed correctly, as described, the etched enamel surface should have a dull, chalky appearance.

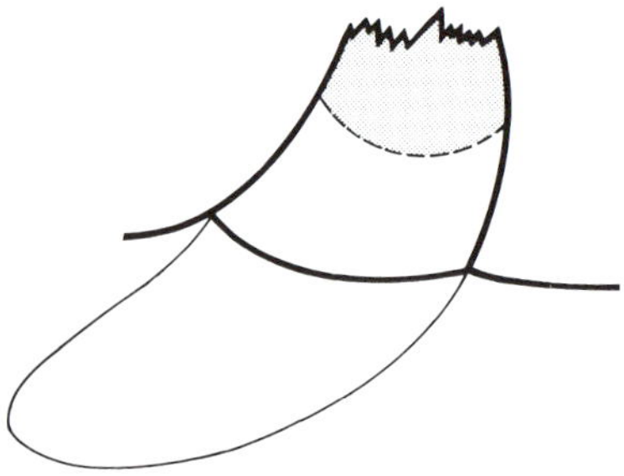

Fig. 7–2. Schematic view of adhesive restoration with etching of the clean enamel surface below the fracture.

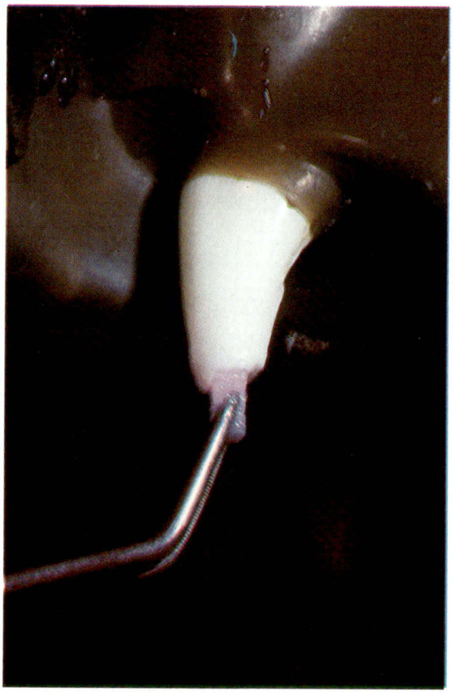

Fig. 7–3. Etching of the enamel surface.

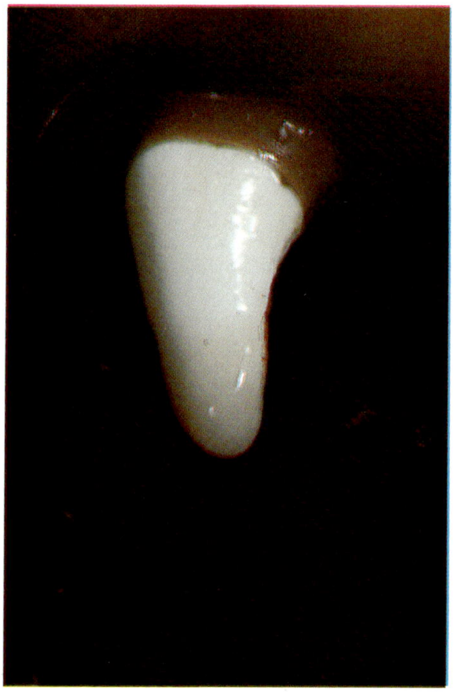

Fig. 7–4. Finished adhesive restoration.

Glossy spots on the etched enamel surface indicate a high fluoride concentration and must be etched again; fluorine hydroxy apatite has a high resistance to acids.

No saliva is allowed to drop onto the etched area, which must not be touched. Microscopically, small points of the etched enamel prisms essential for micromechanical anchorage of the composite can be damaged by saliva or by slight pressure. Composite can now be applied to the etched enamel surface (Fig. 7–4).

One-Phase Technique

Only composites of a pasty consistency are used. Two pastes must be mixed and applied onto the etched enamel surface. The application and modeling of the composite may be done with a plastic spatula or with wet fingers.

Two-Phase Technique

The two-phase technique is recommended for the less-experienced practitioner because the viscosity of the composite can be varied according to one's level of skill. The liquid compounds of the composite are mixed and are applied to the etched enamel and fracture surfaces. Because of the low viscosity of the compounds, a thorough soaking of the enamel pores is guaranteed. Composite paste is then mixed and applied. Liquid composite and composite paste are compatible and can be mixed. By varying the amount of liquid or paste compounds, any desired viscosity can be produced.

Mode of Application

Composite is mixed to a creamy consistency and is applied in layers. At room temperature, hardening of the single layers takes 3 to 5 minutes. The next layer is then applied. If the composite is touched during polymerization, it may break later. To enhance resistance to abrasion, the last layer should be a paste compound. When the last layer is hard, the restoration can be modeled with rotary instruments. A high-speed diamond barrel is useful for this purpose. Abrasives and composite disks in the angle handpiece can be used as well. The more pointed and longer the modeled crown, the more easily it can break. Occlusion should be checked, and if necessary, the antagonist tooth should be trimmed. The owner should prevent the dog from biting hard objects, such as bones, sticks, and stones; normal activity will not affect the restoration. Composites can withstand forces up to 3500 kg/cm^2, equal to the masticatory force in the molar region of large breeds of dogs, such as Rottweilers and Alsatians. After modeling, the restoration can be sealed with a glazing varnish.

The advantage of the acid-etch technique is that it leaves a smooth surface and allows less tartar to form. The disadvantage is that its resistance to abrasion lasts only 4 to 8 months.

ROOT-CANAL POST RESTORATION

Root-canal restoration begins with endodontic treatment, as described in Chapter 6. The tooth stump is then abraded with a pear-head bur on all sides, to ensure that the composite will adhere to the dental neck later. A metal pin of appropriate dimensions is cemented into the root canal. The crown restoration is performed in layers around the pin (Fig. 7–5). This method of crown resto-

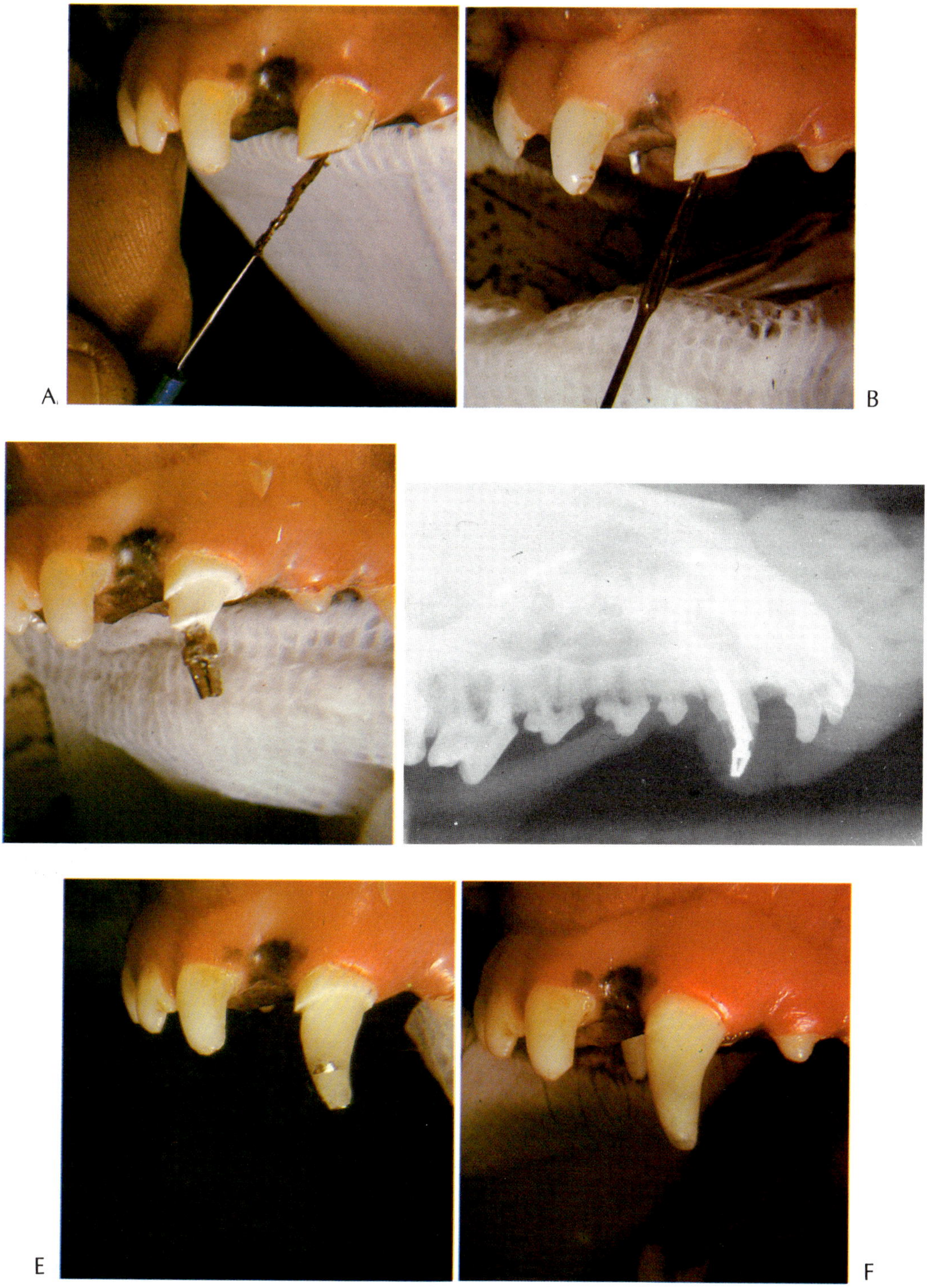

Fig. 7–5. *A,* Pulp extraction. *B,* Enlargement of the root canal. *C,* Metal pin fixation in root-canal phosphate cement. *D,* Radiograph of the repaired tooth. *E,* Metal pin coated partially with composite. *F,* Finished restoration with root-canal post.

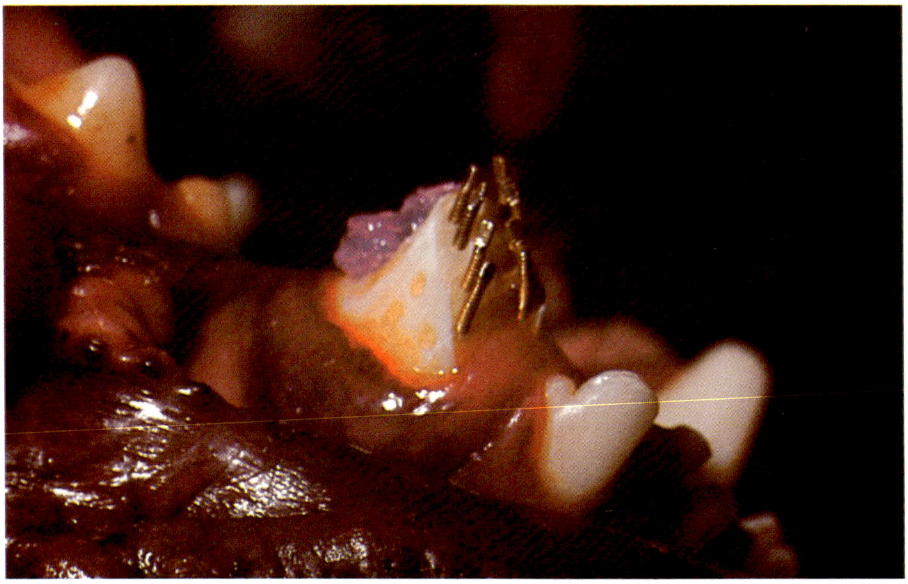

A

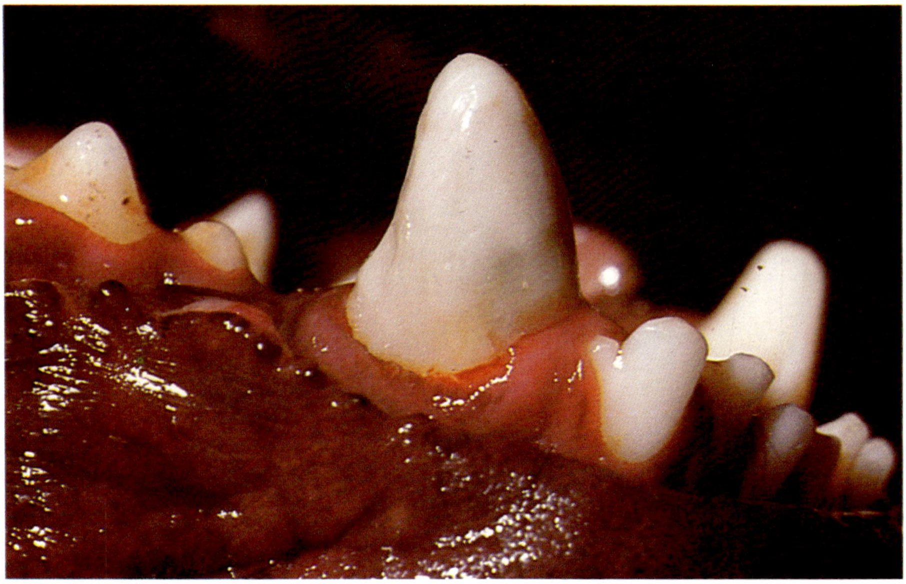

B

Fig. 7–6. *A,* Canine tooth fracture in a military dog. After endodontic treatment, parapulpar pins are fixed in the dentin and are bent to conform to the intended crown form. The residual enamel is etched with violet etching gel. *B,* Finished restoration.

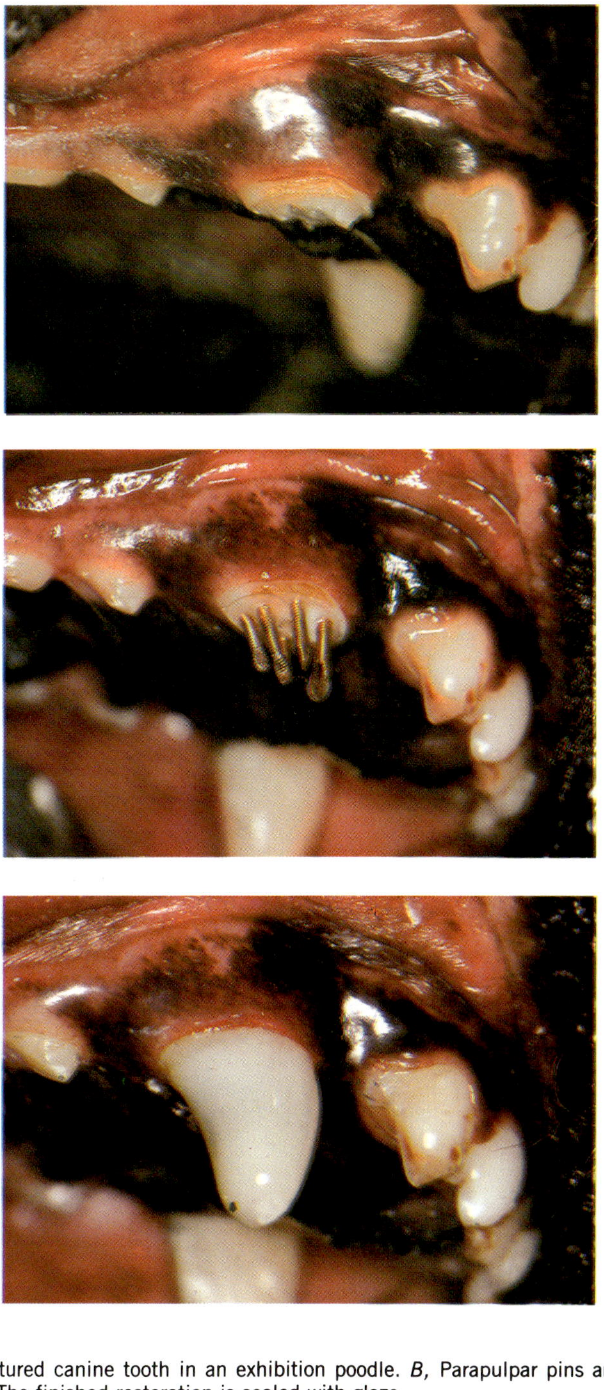

A

B

C

Fig. 7–7. *A*, Fractured canine tooth in an exhibition poodle. *B*, Parapulpar pins are fixed near the enamel margin. *C*, The finished restoration is sealed with glaze.

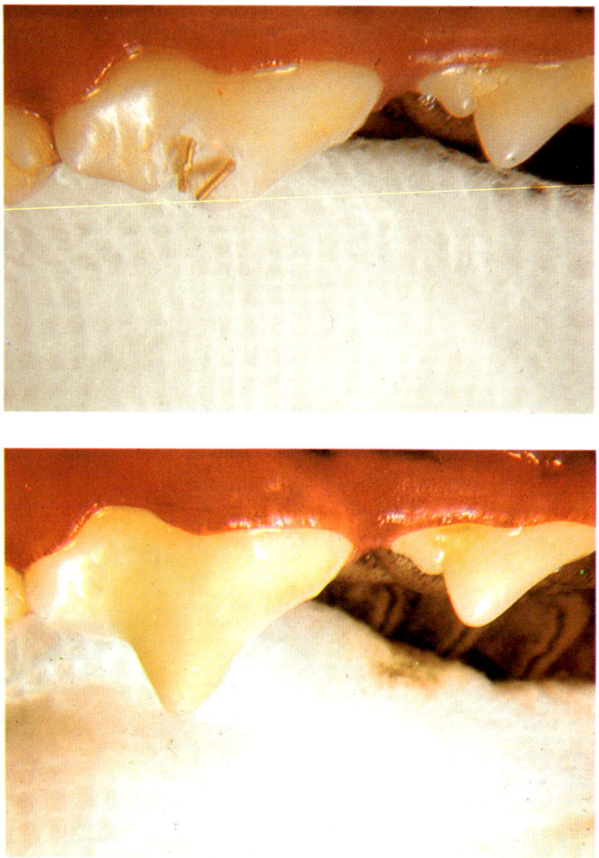

A

B

Fig. 7–8. *A,* Parapulpar pins fixed in the dentin of a fractured P4 in a dog. *B,* Finished restoration.

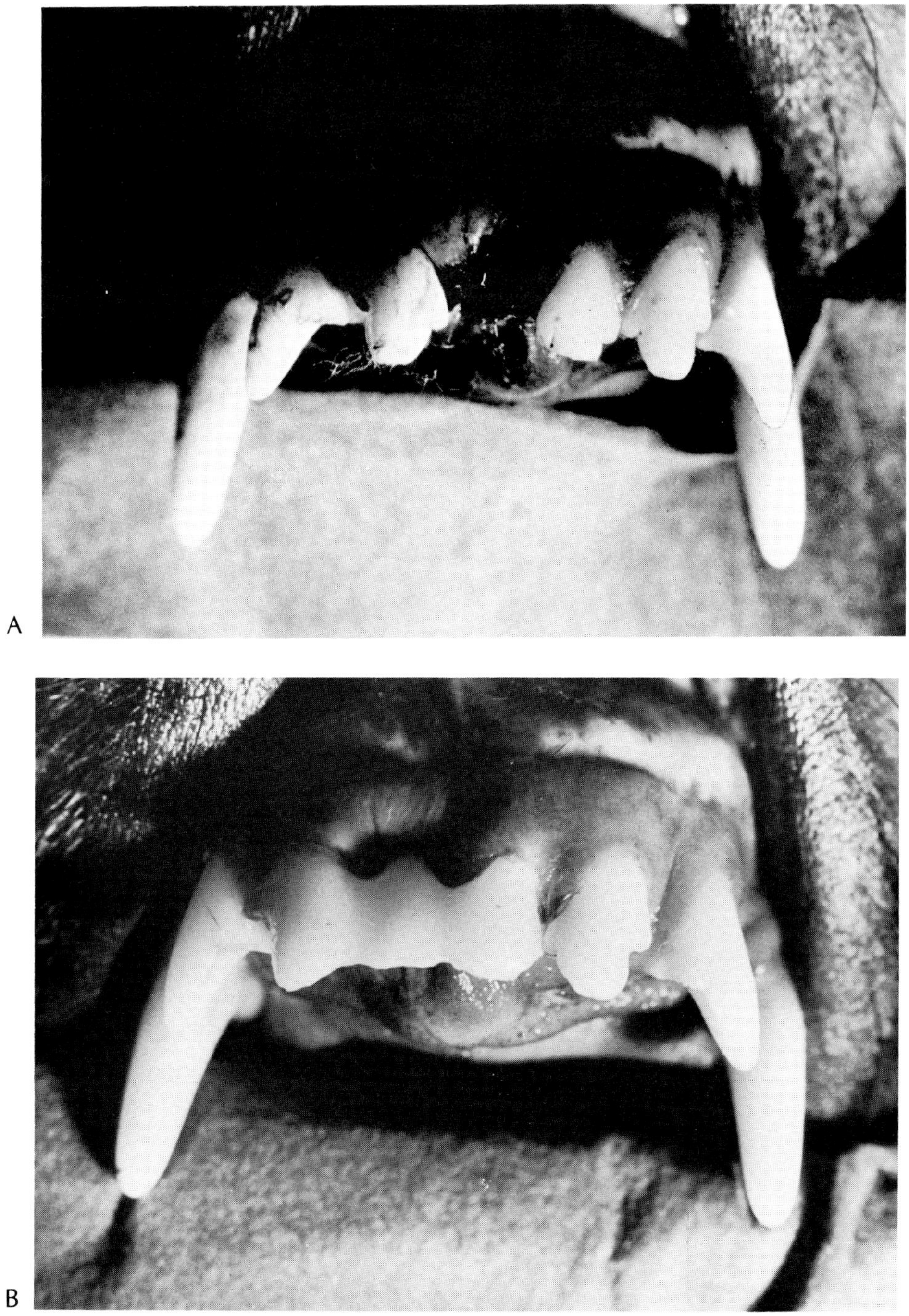

Fig. 7–9. *A,* Traumatic loss of an incisor in a dog. *B,* Cementing of an artificial tooth onto the adjacent teeth by the acid etch technique.

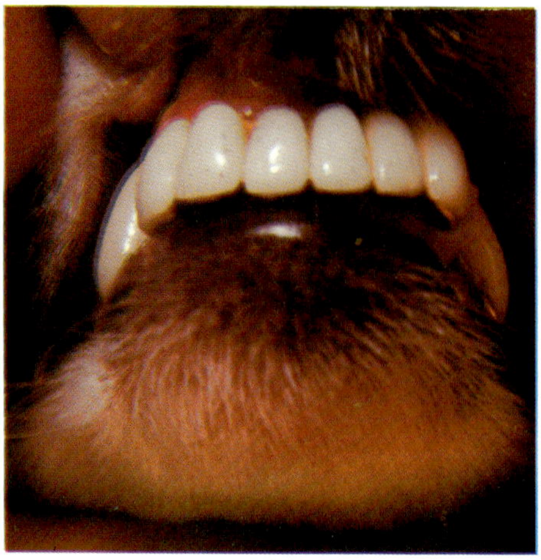

Fig. 7–10. Total incisor denture, cast of gold with porcelain anterior surfaces.

ration is ineffective in larger breeds of dogs because the occlusal forces are too great and force out the pin.

Root canal posts with a mounted crown have excellent mechanical properties; however, because a dental laboratory must prepare the crown, the procedure may be costly.

RESTORATION WITH PARAPULPAR PINS

Additional anchoring of the restoration with parapulpar pins is advisable if sufficient retention can be achieved by the enamel-etch technique (see Fig. 7–7*A*).

Technique

TMS pins adapted for veterinary purposes produce the best results. When the tooth surface has been cleaned parapulpar holes are drilled into the dentin with standardized drills the same size as the pins to be used. The holes should be drilled about 1 mm from the enamel margin, but not in the pulp or the pulp cavity. The depth of the holes should be 2 to 3 mm. The drill should be firmly held to ensure a precisely drilled and centric hole; otherwise, the hole will be too wide, and the pins will loosen.

According to the breed of the patient and the size of the tooth, two to ten pins are used. Gold plated TMS pins are inserted into the parapulpar canals. They have a self-cutting thread and offer the greatest rotational stability. If the pulp is injured accidentally when one is drilling the hole, the pin to be inserted into that particular hole must be coated with a pulp-capping agent. All the pins must be bent to conform to the intended crown shape (Figs. 7–6 and 7–8*A*).

Composite Restoration

Any residual enamel must be prepared for the enamel-etch technique (cleaning, etching, spraying, and drying). Composite should be applied in the same way as in adhesive restoration. The first layer around the pins should have the consistency of whipped cream, which will not alter the shape of the pins as the composite is applied. The best aesthetic results are achieved when the first layer is mixed with an opaquer, so the gold-plated pins cannot be seen through the finished restoration (Figs. 7–6, 7–7, and 7–8).

Once the composite has hardened, it is shaped by grinding, polishing, and sealing in the way described earlier; however, one must be careful when grinding not to touch the parapulpar pins. The restored tooth should not be too long or too sharply pointed; these characteristics increase fragility. Too massive a restoration may affect occlusion; in such a case, it is better to trim the antagonist than to weaken the restoration.

CROWNS

Crowns of cast steel or gold can be used to reconstruct fractured teeth. The tooth stump is prepared as described in Chapter 4, but without grinding any grooves. A dental impression is made and is sent to the dental laboratory. The prefabricated crown is fixed to the stump with phosphate cement. The disadvantages of this therapy are that several visits are necessary, large amounts of anesthesia are used, and the cost is high.

DENTAL BRIDGES

Restoration with Composite and Acid-Etch Technique

Missing teeth in the incisor region can be replaced by prostheses cemented onto the adjacent teeth (Fig. 7–9). Well suited for prosthetic use are the lost tooth, a similar tooth from a different dog, or a tooth modeled from composite paste.

Technique

The enamel surface of the adjacent teeth is prepared by the acid-etch technique. The artificial tooth is fixed in the interdental spaces with composite. After hardening of the temporary fixation, the three teeth are connected by a labial, and if possible palatal, composite bar, which can easily be modeled with a spatula (Fig. 7–9*B*).

Partial Denture with Bridge Construction

A bridge can be constructed to fix loose teeth or to replace lost teeth.

Technique

The abutment teeth are prepared as if for treatment of enamel hypoplasia, but without retention grooves (see Chap. 4). A plaster model of the patient's dentition is made (see Chap. 5). In a dental laboratory, the bridge is cast of gold, with anterior surfaces of plastic or porcelain (Fig. 7–10).

This treatment requires several visits and extensive use of anesthesia; it is also expensive. The dental laboratory must be experienced in veterinary dentistry.

If a vacuum adaptor is at hand, a bridge of transparent acrylic resin that contains the replacement tooth or teeth can be made by the experienced practitioner. The bridge is cemented onto the abutment teeth by the acid-etch technique (Fig. 7–11).

Bibliography: 6, 9, 15, 18, 31, 39, 57, 62

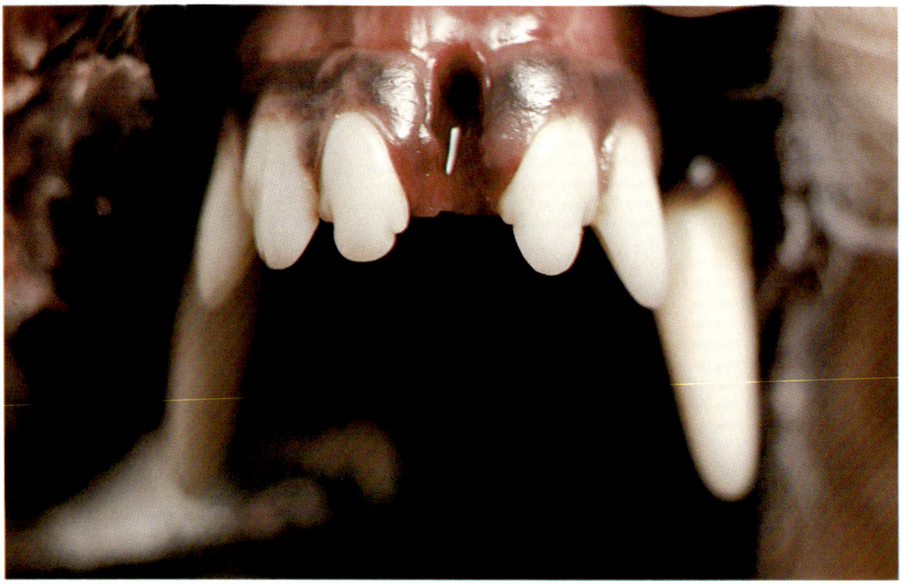

A

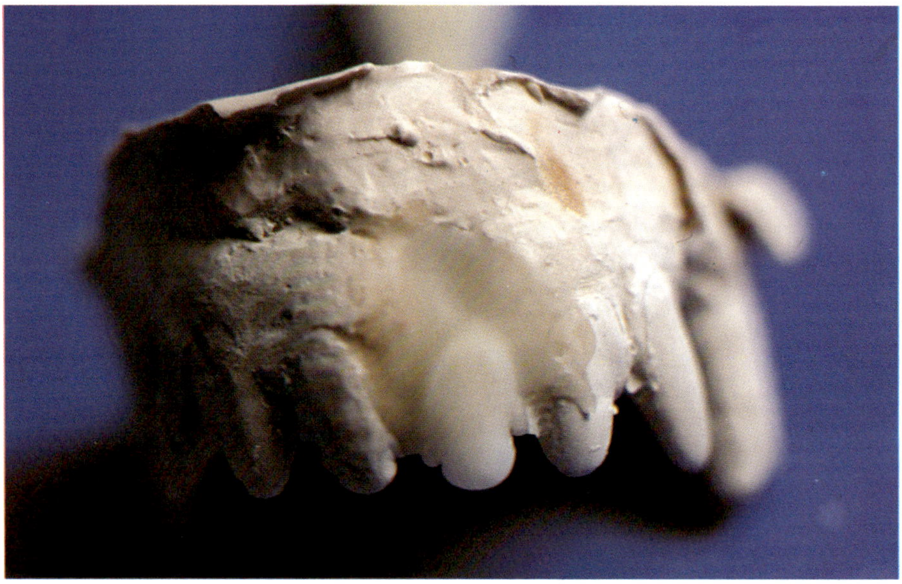

B

Fig. 7–11. *A,* Traumatic loss of I1 in a dog. *B,* The lost tooth, without its roots, is embedded in wax on a plaster model.

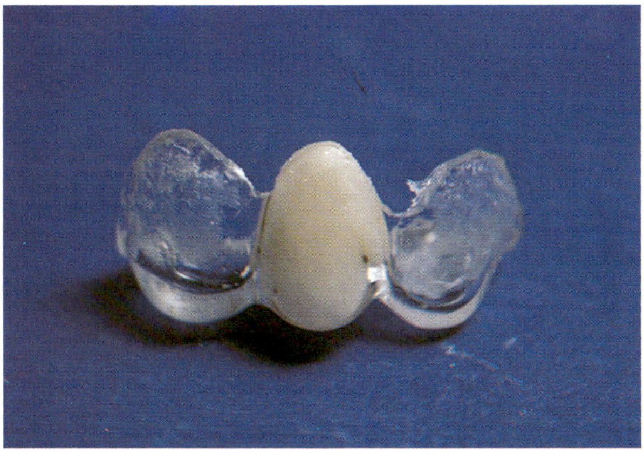

A

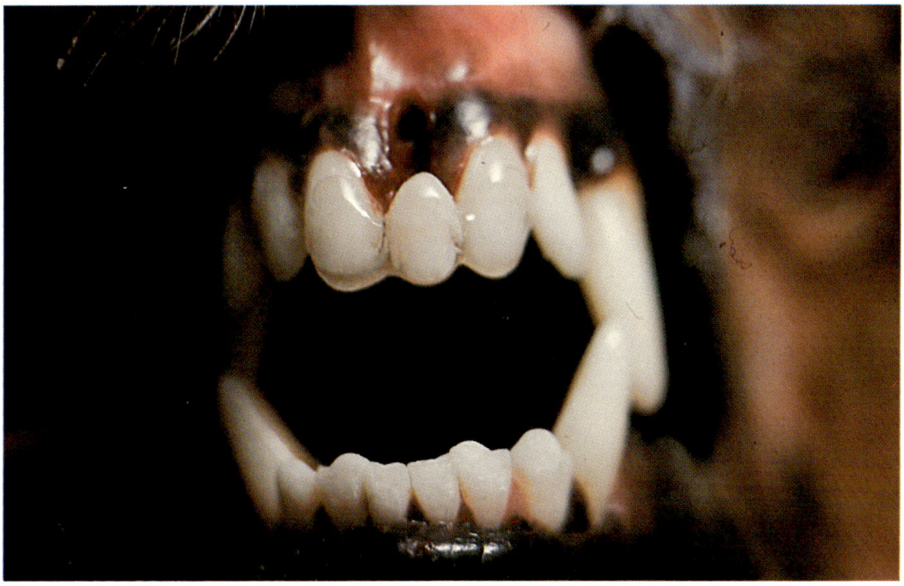

B

Fig. 7–11. ***Continued*** *C,* Bridge of acrylic resin made in a vacuum adaptor; the dog's lost tooth has been inserted in the bridge. *D,* The bridge is cemented onto the adjacent teeth by the acid etch technique.

8

Caries

Caries, a demineralization of the hard tooth substance, is caused by bacterial acid production. We distinguish among crown, neck, and root caries. Morphologically speaking, caries can be superficial, deep, or penetrating (to the opening of the pulp cavity). Caries in dogs develop faster than those in herbivores. The decalcification of enamel is initiated by cariogenic plaque bacteria that produce acids from carbohydrates. Proteolytic enzymes of different kinds of bacteria destroy the exposed organic components of the tooth substance. Both processes enhance the spreading of caries in the soft dentin.

Caries in carnivores occur rarely, by comparison with herbivores and omnivores, for the following reasons: the food of carnivores contains few cariogenic components, such as carbohydrates; the cariogenic acid producers *Streptococcus mutans* and *S. salivarius*, which are typical human plaque flora, are not found in carnivores; most teeth in carnivores are cone-shaped, so the approximal sur-

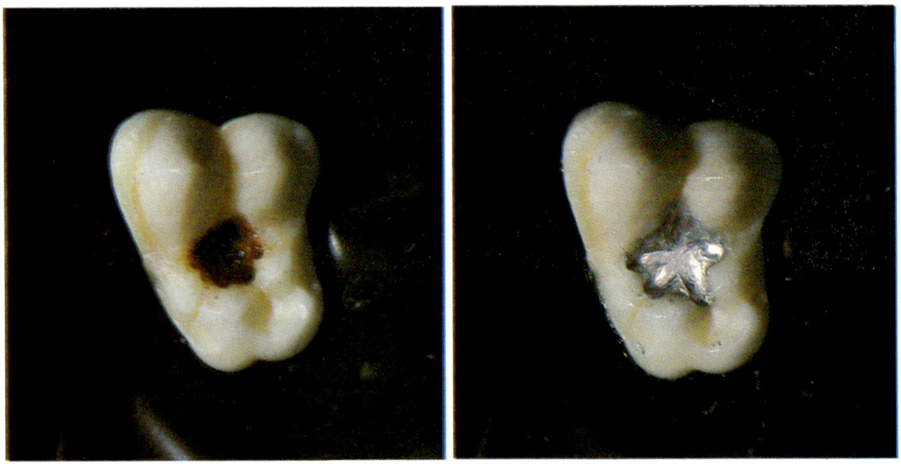

A B

Fig. 8–1. *A*, Central pit caries of maxillary M1 in a dog. The tooth is isolated by a rubber dam. *B*, Silver amalgam filling. The fissures of the occlusal surface must be prepared carefully to avoid secondary fissure caries.

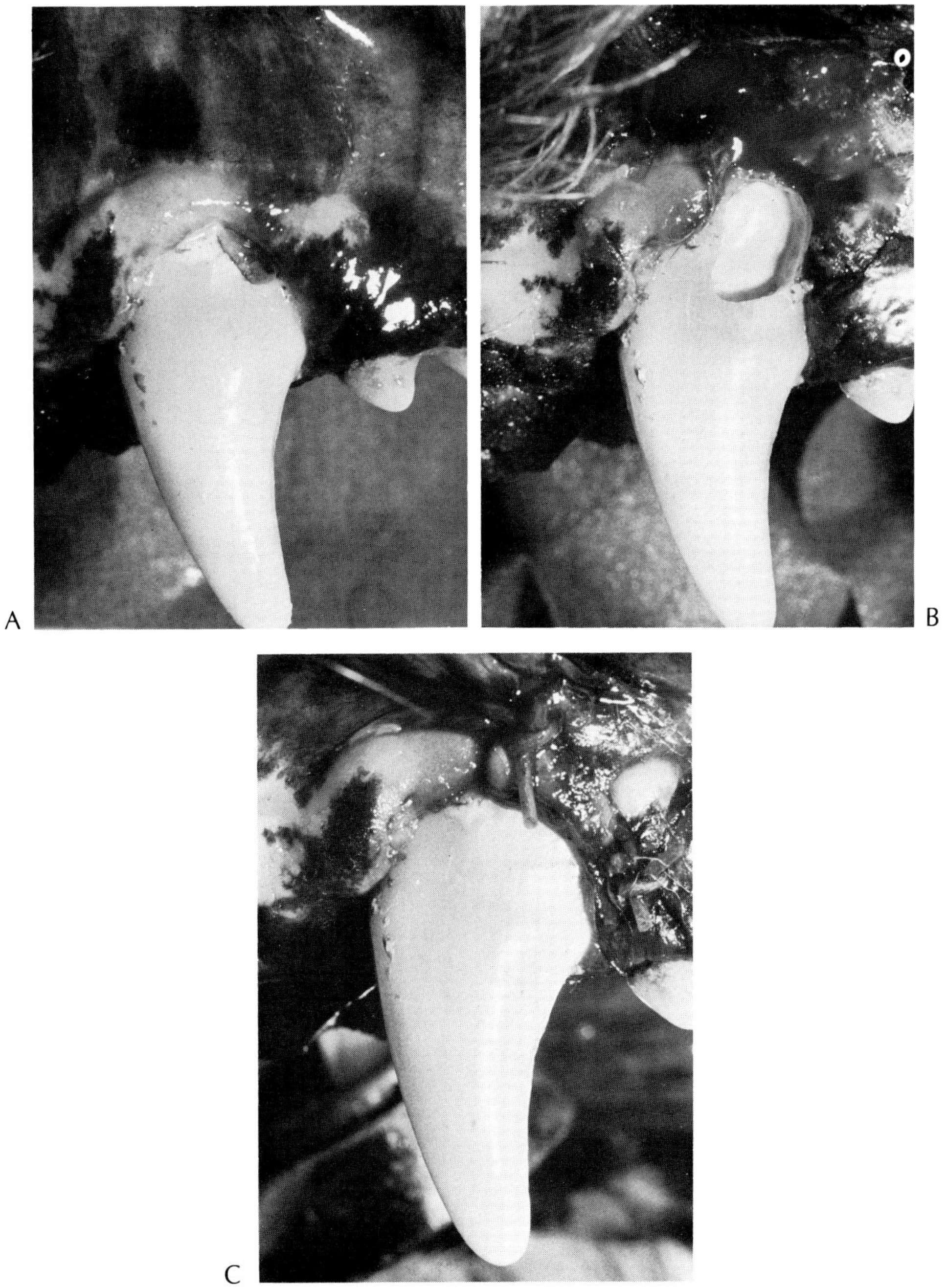

Fig. 8–2. Neck caries of a canine tooth in a dog. *A,* The lesion extends subgingivally. *B,* The whole extent of the carious lesion can be seen after lifting a gingival flap; the cavity has been prepared and sealed with cavity liner. *C,* Filling with composite. The gingival flap has been repositioned and sutured with chromic catgut.

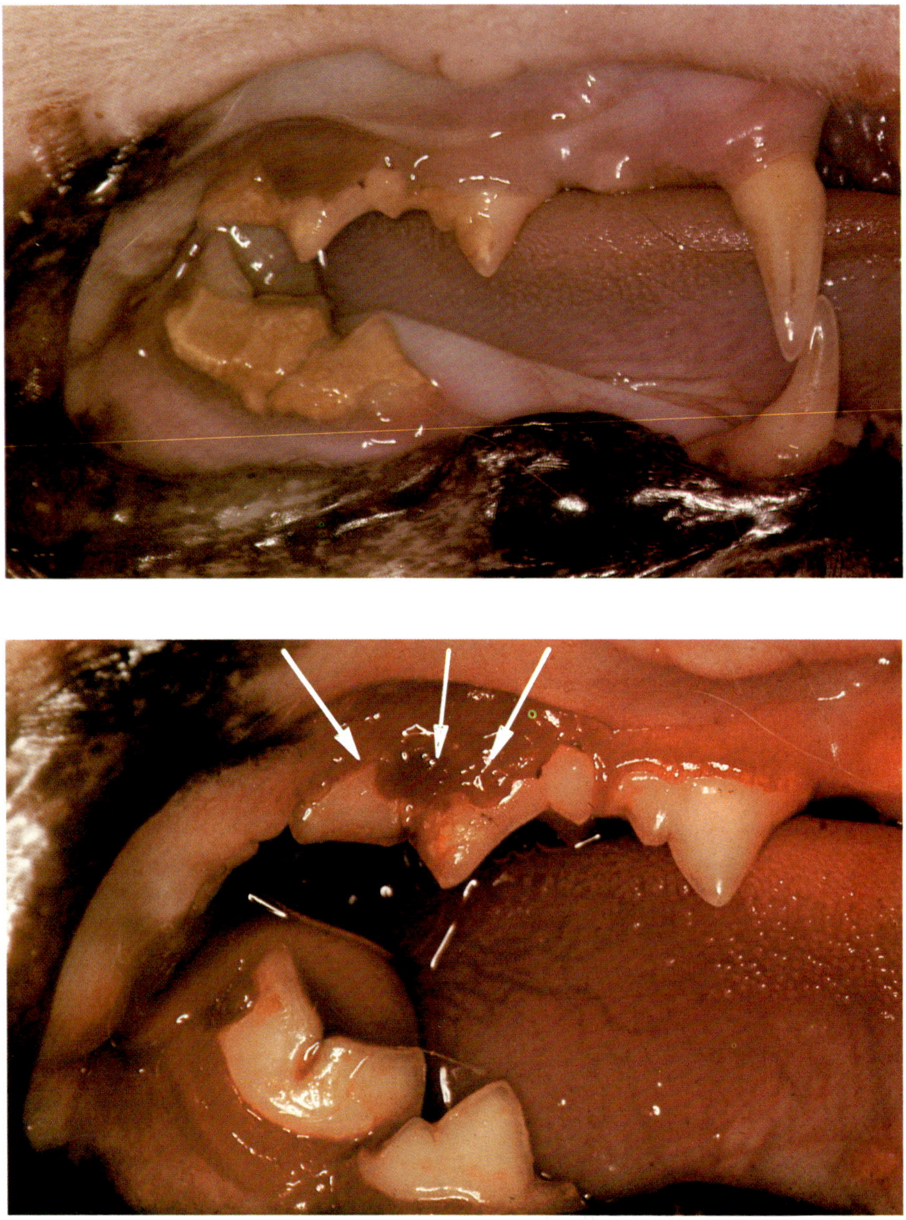

A

B

Fig. 8–3. Neck lesions in a cat. *A,* Plaque and tartar cover most of the lesions in the upper and lower jaw. *B,* When the tooth surfaces have been cleaned, the lesions, filled with granulation tissue (arrows), become visible.

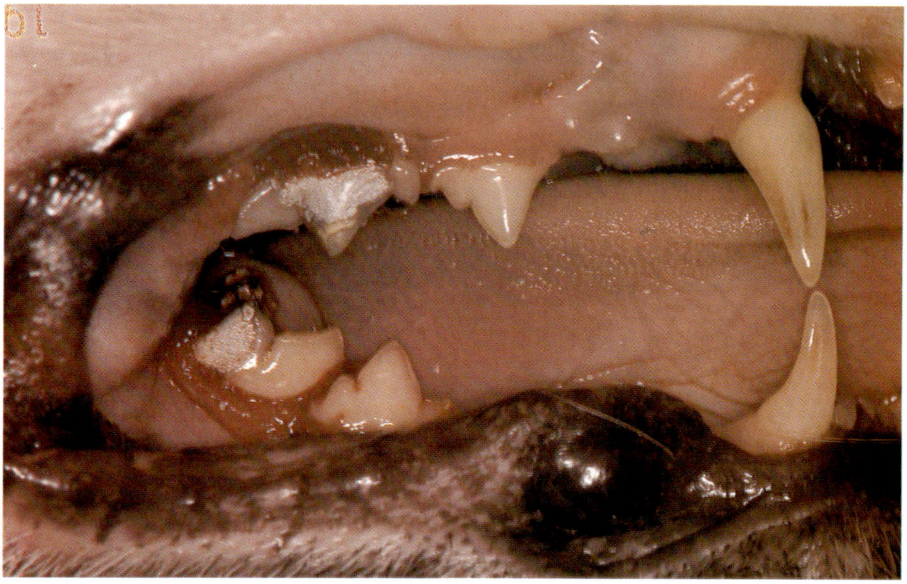

C

Fig. 8–3. ***Continued*** *C,* After endodontic treatment, the cavities are filled with normal silver amalgam.

faces and the pits and fissures that are the retention sites for bacteria and food debris in human teeth do not exist, except in the individual molars (Fig. 8–1). It is not known whether immune globulins in the saliva of carnivores play a part in resistance to caries. Breed, individual constitution, and diet contribute to the incidence of caries. Caries are common in cats, and a genetic disposition to caries has been observed in purebred cats.

The shape and function of teeth in primates are similar to those in man, and caries occur often. The teeth of cattle and pigs are prone to caries, but one does not need to treat them because of the short life span of these animals. Caries in horses may occur in connection with cementum hypoplasia of the molars.

PREDILECTION SITES

Dogs

Caries occur in the central pits of the maxillary M1 (Fig. 8–1) and the necks of the canine teeth (Fig. 8–2), as well as in the region of the gingival pockets.

Cats

The necks of the canines, premolars, and molars are most commonly affected (Fig. 8–3).

Herbivores

In these animals, one may see cavities of hypoplastic molars.

SIGNS AND SYMPTOMS

Brown to grayish brown or black discoloring and softening of hard dental substance are signs of caries. The caries contain bacteria and food debris and give off a characteristic odor. The hard, resistant enamel margins are less directly affected than the dentin, so the dentinal lesion is larger than the visible opening. Pain is produced by the penetration of bacterial toxins and chemical irritants into the dentinal tubules. In direct consequence, pulpitis develops, eventually leading to pulp necrosis or periapical granuloma. In cats, the caries do not show a brown discoloration and softening of dentin. The lesion starts from the tooth neck and spreads until the tooth is hollow and breaks. Sharp points remain and are often the cause of untreatable gingivitis and periodontitis.

TREATMENT

See "Preparing the Tooth" in Chapter 3 for a description of how the carious tooth should be prepared for treatment. It is essential to extend the preparation of the central pit caries of the maxillary M1 in the dog into the fissures, to prevent the formation of secondary fissure caries. To recognize the full extent of the canine neck caries, it is often advisable to lift a gingival flap (see Fig. 8–2*B*).

In cats, the cavity is prepared with the continuous use of the air blower, to keep the area clear of heavily bleeding granulation tissue.

If a sound pulp is injured during preparation, direct pulp capping with calcium hydroxide must be performed, as in vital amputation (see Chap. 6).

In advanced caries, the pulp becomes necrotic, and mortal amputation or pulp extirpation must be performed.

If, after performing cavity preparation, the pulp is visible through the thin dentin layer, indirect pulp capping with calcium hydroxide is recommended.

Permanent filling of cavities is with amalgam or composite (see Figs. 8–1*B*, 8–2*C*, and 8–3*C*).

In cats, normal silver amalgam must be used rather than non-gamma-2 amalgam. It is applied in layers, while continuously using the air blower to prevent bleeding into the cavity. One must not overfill the molars and thereby cause an interference in occlusion, which is recognized by the glossiness of the occlusal surface. Immediately after filling the tooth, occlusion should be checked, and if necessary, the filling should be modeled with a carver. Cats with caries often develop lesions elsewhere and should be checked twice yearly.

Bibliography: 11, 25, 34, 35, 41, 58

9

Periodontal Diseases

These diseases are common in dogs and cats; the knowledge of their pathogenesis and treatment is important for modern small animal practice. At the end of this chapter is a brief discussion of periodontal diseases of rodents and reptiles. Alveolar inflammation in horses is different in origin and treatment from these diseases and is described in Chapter 6.

GINGIVITIS, PERIODONTITIS, PLAQUE, AND TARTAR

Origin

Most inflammatory diseases of the gingiva and periodontium are caused by a formation of mycotic and bacterial deposits, or plaque, on the tooth surface. Gingiva and periodontium are irritated by bacterial toxins. The term gingivitis is used for an inflammation of the gingival tissue, whereas periodontitis involves an advanced inflammation of deeper tissue layers.

Plaque deposits can be made visible by plaque-disclosing agents. A few drops of sodium fluorescein are distributed over the tooth surfaces and the gingiva; then half a glass of water is poured over the dentition; the sodium fluorescein does not stick to the clean tooth surfaces and gingiva, but adheres to the plaque, mycotic deposits, and necrotic gingiva, which then give off a bright fluorescence when illuminated by blue or ultraviolet light (Fig. 9–1). For scientific documentation, the range of staining can be shown by ultraviolet fluorescence photography.

Pathogenesis

The immunologic system of a sound animal is responsible for an equilibrium between bacterial plaque formation and defense mechanism. An overgrowth of plaque may develop with a decreased defense mechanism in certain breeds of dogs, such as miniature breeds, including the Chihuahua, poodle, Yorkshire terrier, and dachshund. The enzymes of the plaque metabolism (hyaluronidase, collagenase) penetrate the gingiva and soften it (Fig. 9–2). The infiltration of the gingiva with bacteria and high-molecular toxins causes immunologic reactions and formation of antigen-antibody complexes. During the phase of phagocytosis, lysosomal enzymes that can affect or can even destroy the gingival or periodontal

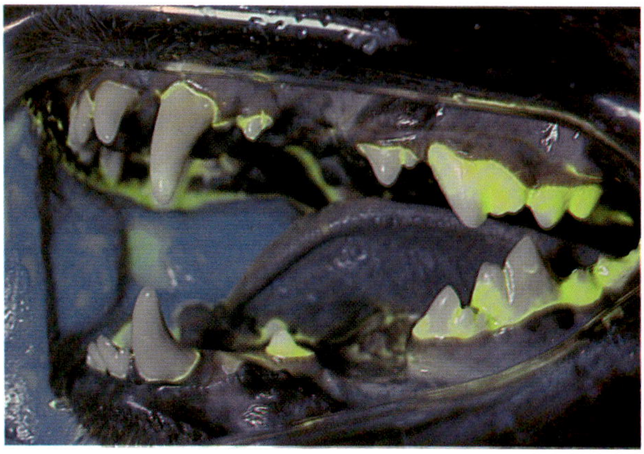

Fig. 9–1. Staining plaque with sodium fluorescein illuminated by blue or ultraviolet light.

tissue may be released. These processes may be intense enough to cause the loosening or even shedding of teeth.

If gingival attachment to tooth and alveolus is lost, gingival pockets will develop (Fig. 9–2*B*). Within these pockets, the self-cleaning mechanisms of the oral cavity, such as salivation and tongue and cheek movements, are not effective. Consequently, subgingival tartar or caries will develop (Fig. 9–2*C*). Plaque deposits are calcified to tartar by the mineral salts of saliva. Tartar is yellow, brown, or dark brown and occurs as a visible supragingival substance or is found in the gingival pockets as a subgingival substance. Subgingival tartar is often stained greenish or green brown by the degradation products of the blood (hemosiderin). It is detrimental because it continuously irritates the inner wall of the pocket with its rough surface; it is often overlooked when removing other tartar. Bacterial irritants and mechanical pressure of the progressively growing subgingival tartar destroy the periodontium toward the root apex and are the main cause for the loosening of teeth (Fig. 9–3).

Supragingival tartar is particularly common on the canine teeth as well as the buccal surfaces of P3, P4, and M1 in the maxilla, where the parotid duct enters the oral cavity. In advanced cases of tartar formation, the loosened M1 in the maxilla is fixed to the adjacent P4 by a so-called "tartar-bridge." Sometimes, a small "fracture line" in the tartar between these two teeth can be noticed (Fig. 9–4). The tartar must be removed, even if M1 is shed in the process.

Between the supragingival tartar margin and receded gingiva, one often sees a furrow filled with malodorous food debris, hairs, bacteria, and necrotic tissue. The underlying gingiva is chronically inflamed and ulcerated and shows a strong tendency to bleed. In older animals, kissing ulcers may occur at those places where the mucosa of the flews or cheek comes into close contact with plaque deposits (Fig. 9–4). Besides bacterial toxins, urease-forming bacteria are responsible for ulceration; these special bacteria decompose the urea, excreted into the oral cavity in cases of chronic renal insufficiency, to ammonia. In cases of advanced tartar formation, tartar is to be found even on the palatal and lingual surfaces. The mandibular molars do not form tartar to such a great extent because of occlusal friction. The mechanical pressure of the continuously formed tartar is responsible for the recession of gingiva and alveolar bone (see Fig. 9–4).

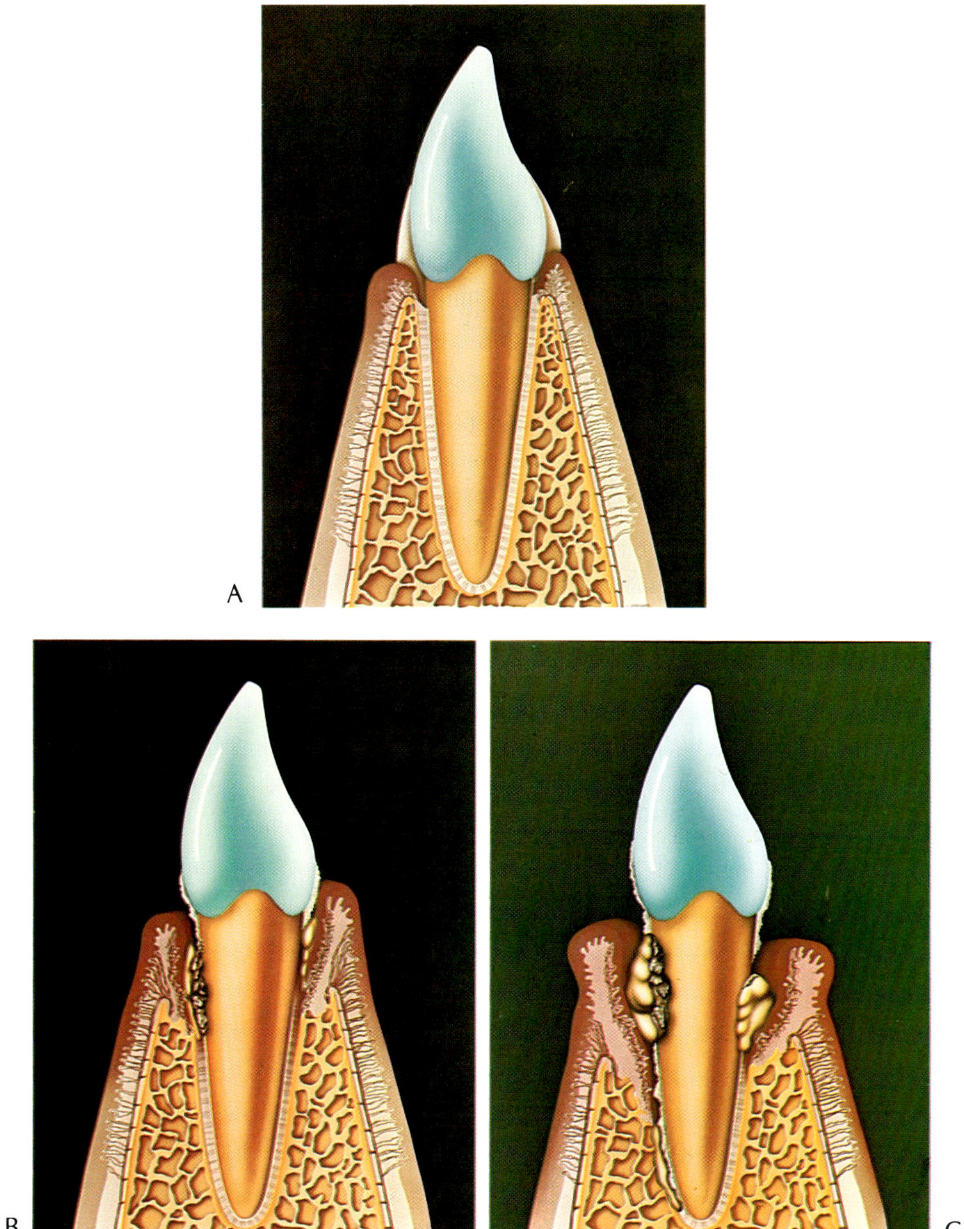

Fig. 9–2. Pathogenesis of periodontal diseases. *A,* Plaque deposit on the neck of a tooth, with marginal gingivitis. *B,* Formation of gingival pockets and subgingival tartar. *C,* Progression of plaque and tartar toward the root apex, with marked swelling and inflammation of the gingiva, loss of gingiva and alveolar bone, and loosening of the tooth.

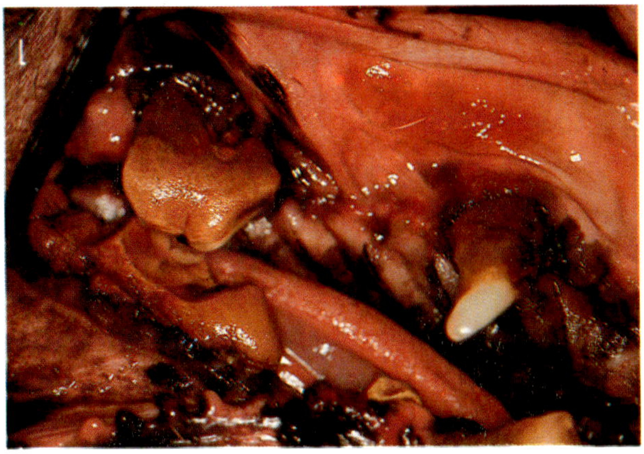

Fig. 9–3. Excessive tartar formation in a dog. The roots of P4 are partially exposed by recession of the gingival and alveolar margins.

Besides these mechanical influences, the foregoing autodestructive immunologic processes play an important part.

Treatment

Whenever possible, a one-week course of antibiotic pretreatment is advisable, to allow tartar removal in an uncontaminated oral cavity. The advantage for the patient is a reduced risk of bacteremia during extensive therapy in the oral cavity. The advantage for the practitioner is a reduced risk of contamination, by inhalation of contaminated spray from the ultrasonic cleaner.

Mechanical Removal of Tartar and Plaque

A thorough treatment of the oral cavity should be performed during a general examination including vaccination, depletion of anal sacs, or cleaning of ears.

Plaque and tartar can be removed with curettes, scalers, and ultrasonic cleaners (see Chap. 3). The straight or curved scaler is moved from the gingival margin

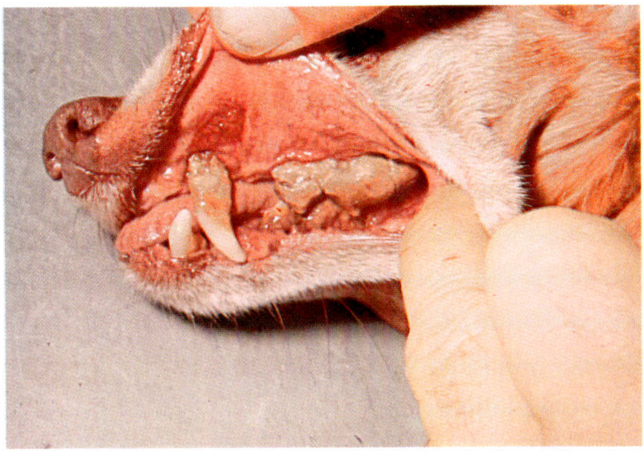

Fig. 9–4. Excessive plaque and tartar formation in a dog. A tartar bridge between the maxillary P4 and the loosened M1 is clearly visible. Kissing ulcers are present on the flews in the canine area.

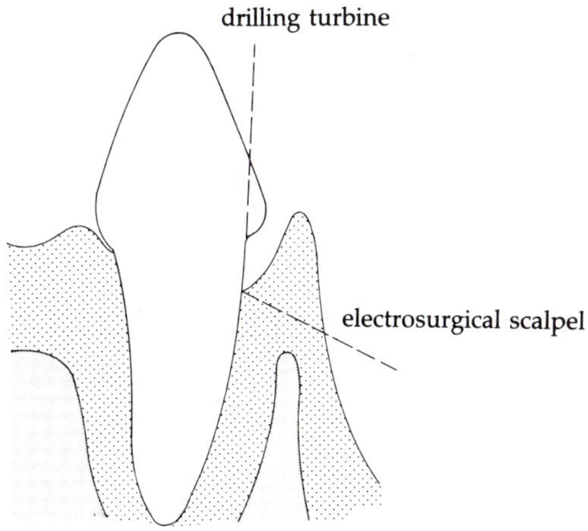

Fig. 9–5. Schematic view of gingivectomy odontoplasty; removal of the enamel ridge on the tooth neck and resection of the gingival pocket (gingivectomy).

toward the crown top. The curved scaler is specially suited for the cleaning of gingival pockets. Loosened teeth should not be cleaned with hand scalers.

For quick, careful, and thorough cleaning, an ultrasonic cleaner should be used. Tuning frequency is less important than reliable water cooling of the vibrating tip. Various tips for ultrasonic cleaners are available; chisel-shaped, broad tips are best.

The ultrasonic cleaner should always be kept in motion, to avoid thermal damage to the tooth surface. The least amount of pressure that will remove calculus is used, to prevent microetching of the enamel. The highest efficiency is achieved when the tip is held at an angle of 45° to the tooth surface. Tartar should also be removed from both the gingival pockets and the lingual and palatal surfaces of the teeth, but not with the ultrasonic scaler. The best instrument to use is the subgingival curette.

Root Planing

When tartar is removed from exposed tooth necks or root portions, a rough surface remains. Such surfaces must be planed carefully to delay tartar and plaque formation (see Fig. 9–6*B*).

The planing instruments should be used in the following order: bullet-shaped diamond in a dental turbine handpiece for coarse planing; composite disks for fine planing; scalers for approximal surfaces, such as between maxillary P4 and M1; and rubber polishers for finishing, using an abrasive dental prophylaxis paste.

Odontoplasty

The tooth neck in small animals has an enamel ridge about 1 to 2 mm high surrounding the whole tooth; in some teeth, the gingiva is inserted into this ridge. In cases of gingival recession, plaque and food debris readily collect in the furrow between the ridge and the gingiva (see Fig. 9–6*A*). Removal of this enamel ridge enhances the self-cleaning mechanism of the teeth (Figs. 9–5 and 9–6).

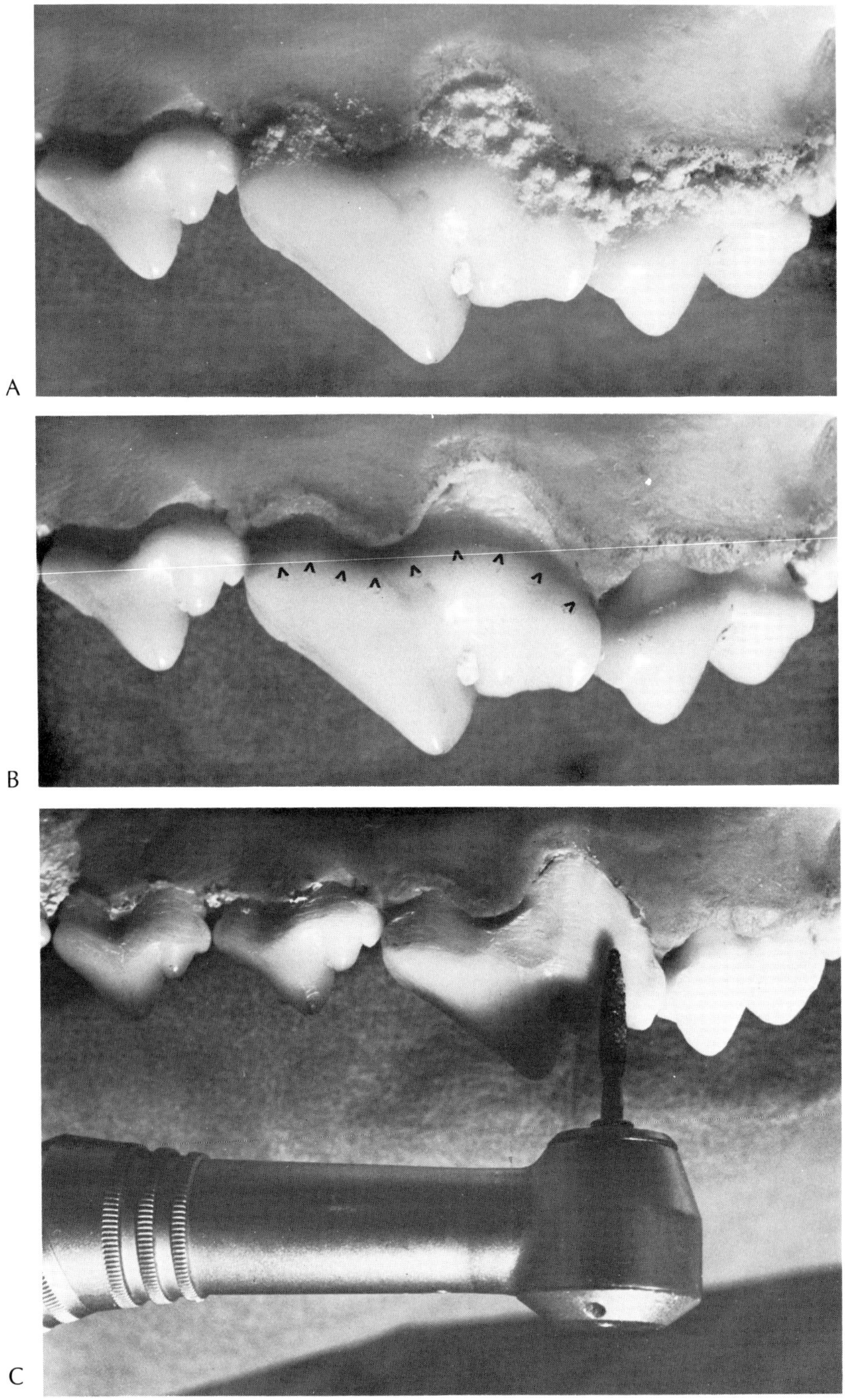

Fig. 9–6. Odontoplasty and root planing. *A,* Formation of plaque and tartar between the enamel ridge and the receded gingival margin. *B,* After removing the plaque and tartar, the rough root surface and the enamel ridge *(arrows)* around the tooth become visible. *C,* The enamel ridge is trimmed to enhance the self-cleaning mechanism of the teeth.

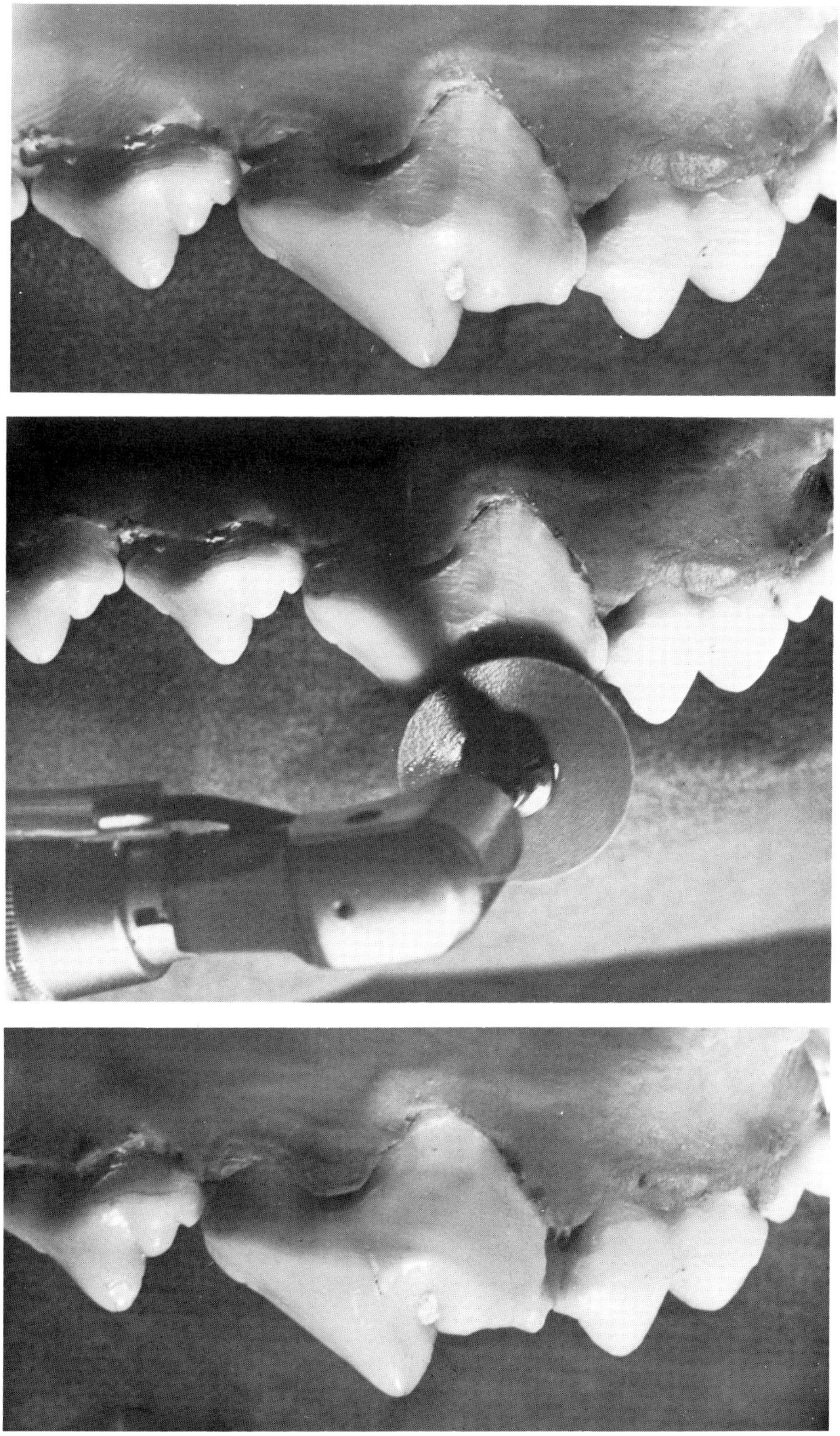

D

E

F

Fig. 9–6. ***Continued*** *D*, After trimming, the diamond barrel leaves tiny grooves. *E*, The rough surfaces are planed with composite disks and rubber polishers. *F*, The formation of bacterial deposits and tartar will be delayed on the smooth surfaces of the tooth and root.

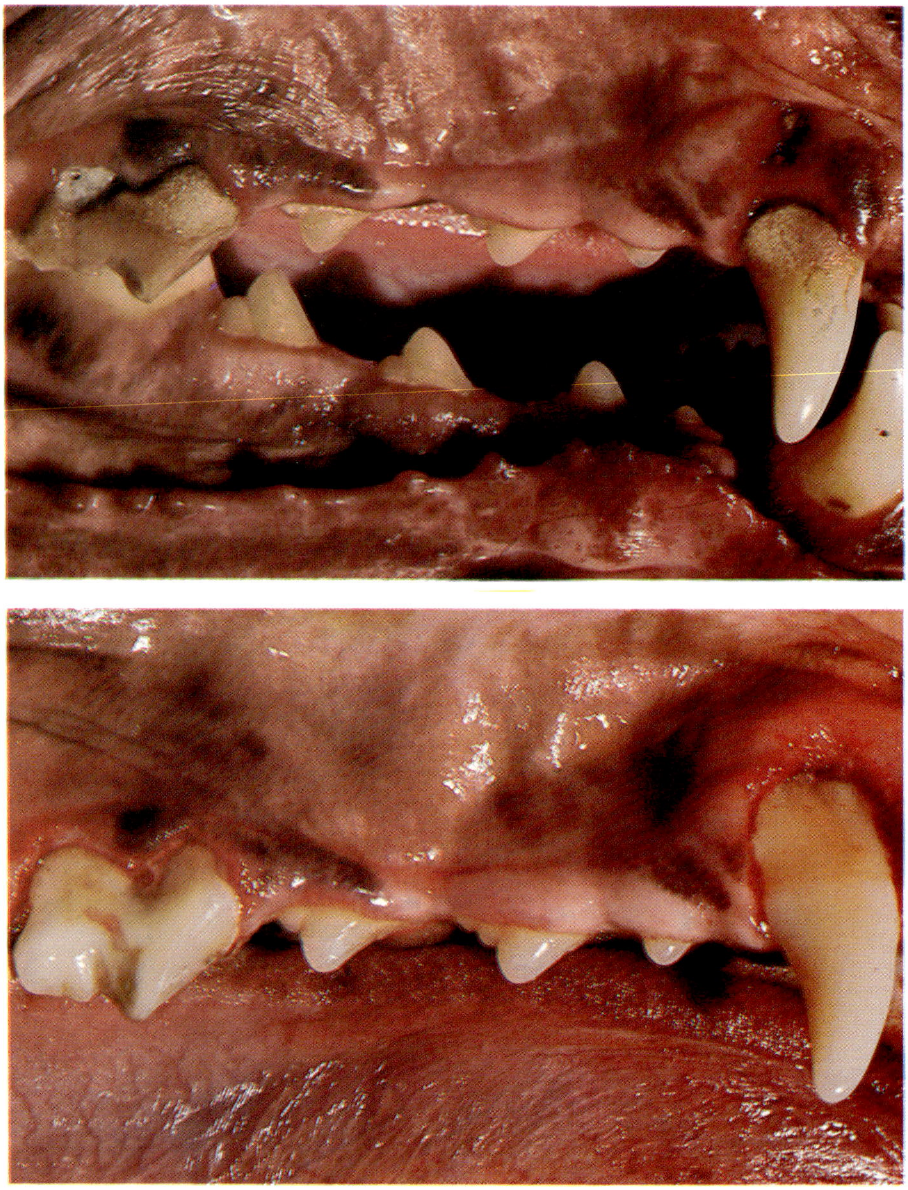

A

B

Fig. 9–7. *A,* Plaque, tartar, pocket formation, and gingival recession are clearly visible in P4 and M1. *B,* The same teeth after external gingivectomy, root planing, and odontoplasty.

C 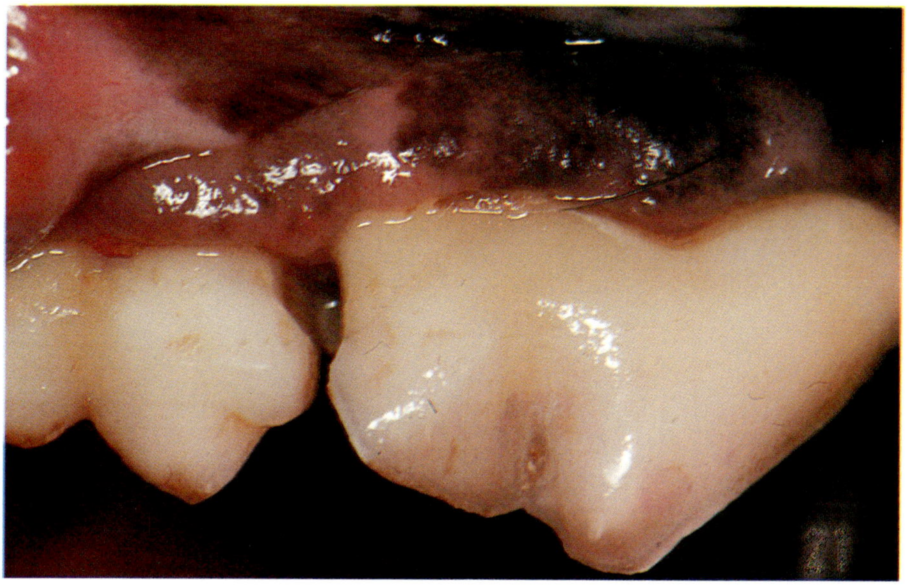

Fig. 9–7. ***Continued*** *C*, Follow-up a year after the operation; regular tooth brushing by the owner has maintained excellent hygiene.

The appropriate instruments are a diamond barrel or fissure bur and abrasives in the angle handpiece.

Technique. The enamel ridge is removed on the buccal, and if necessary even on the labial, surface with rotary instruments. The contact point between two adjacent teeth must not be trimmed off, particularly the point between the maxillary P4 and M1. The contact point forms a ridge that retains the teeth. After trimming, one should check the surface for smoothness. The diamond instrument leaves tiny grooves that accelerate the reaccumulation of tartar. These grooves must be polished with composite disks and rubber polishers (Fig. 9–6).

Gingivectomy

Subgingival tartar, which is revealed on resecting the gingiva, can then be completely removed along with any possible remnants of bacterial aggregations.

The instruments used for gingivectomy are an electrosurgery unit and scalpel or special gingivectomy instruments.

Technique. For the less-experienced practitioner, we recommend putting small needle holes in the gingiva, to create small bleeding points that mark the pocket depth. The detached gingiva is then removed by an oblique incision to the bottom of the pocket (Figs. 9–5 and 9–7). Both ends of the incision should be shallow, to avoid cutting the corners or edges of the tooth.

The high-frequency voltage of the electrosurgery unit should be regulated in such a way that, on the one hand, the incision can be performed uniformly and, on the other hand, no sparks are discharged.

The electrode should not come into contact with bone; bone necrosis could result.

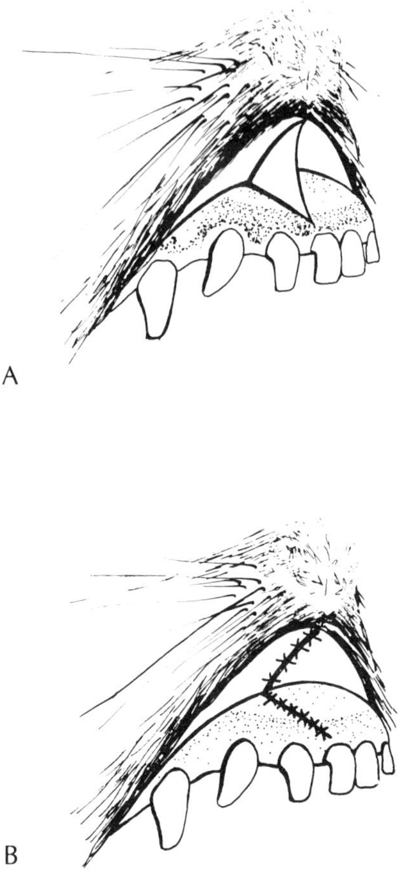

Fig. 9–8. *A* and *B*, Spindle-shaped frenectomy.

Frenectomy

In certain cases, the hypoplastic frenulum causes the gingiva to be under abnormally strong pressure. Local gingival recession can thereby occur.

Three important frenula are present in dogs. One of these is situated between the lip and the central incisors in the maxilla (Fig. 9–8*A*). The second and third frenula occur between the labial surfaces of the canine teeth and the anterior part of the flews in the mandible.

Technique. In some cases, subgingival dissection of the collagenous fibers is sufficient. In most cases, a spindle-shaped excision of the frenulum is indicated (Fig. 9–8*B*). Exceptional apical displacement of the gingival attachment is useful for the mandibular frenula: the frenulum is dissected close to the gingival margin, and the detached labial mucosa of the flews is apically displaced and is sutured to the periosteum. Gingival recession is stopped because of the absence of tensile forces.

Gingivoplasty

Chronic gingivitis may lead to proliferation or thickening of marginal gingiva, particularly in certain breeds of dogs, such as boxers, collies, and afghan hounds. Dissecting marginal proliferations at an acute angle enhances the self-cleaning

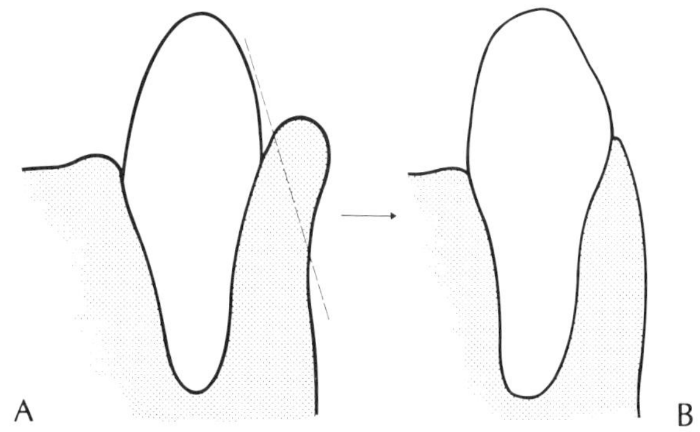

Fig. 9–9. *A* and *B*, Gingivoplasty. Note the acute angle of incision *(A)*.

mechanism of the oral cavity and deflects food from the vulnerable region of gingival insertion (Fig. 9–9). The electrosurgery unit is recommended for this purpose because the operation can be performed almost without bleeding.

Cautious topical application with a cotton swab of 50% trichloracetic acid solution is recommended, especially in cats, as a kind of "chemical gingivoplasty."

Flap Surgery

If the incisors are slightly loosened as well as covered by plaque and tartar, a flap operation can enhance self-cleaning in this region, as well as stabilizing the teeth.

Gingival pockets that extend beyond the mucogingival line are an indication for this type of operation. The mucogingival line, present between the attached gingiva and the freely movable mucosa, can easily be recognized as a notched, thin, red line (see Fig. 9–7*A* and *B*).

The presence of bony pockets or bony proliferations at the alveolar crest is also an indication for flap procedure.

Technique. A vertical incision is made through the mucosa and the periosteum (Fig. 9–10*A*). The position of the vertical incision depends on the width of the mucoperiosteal flap. When one has dissected the marginal gingiva by internal gingivectomy, the mucoperiosteal flap can be lifted with a periosteal elevator.

Exposed root surfaces should be thoroughly cleaned and polished. Bone form is corrected with chisels, burs, or diamond barrels (Fig. 9–10*B*). This kind of correction is commonly called osteoplasty, that is, trimming alveolar bone and recreating a functional form.

Necrotic remnants of gingiva should be removed; bony pockets should be eliminated by planing the alveolar bone contour. The purpose of all such corrections is to create a shallow and gentle form of the bone surfaces that soft tissue can follow.

The flap is repositioned and interdentally sutured (Fig. 9–10C). According to our experience, surgical dressings are not advantageous in the healing process. If used, preparations must be mixed according to the manufacturers' instructions and then applied to the teeth and gingiva. The hardened pack is removed in 4 to 7 days.

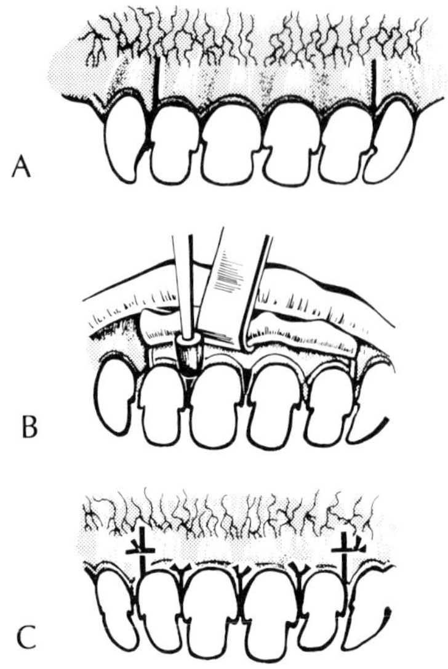

Fig. 9–10. Schematic view of flap operation. *A*, Vertical incisions. *B*, Osteoplasty of the exposed alveolar ridge and polishing of exposed root surfaces. *C*, Repositioning of the mucoperiosteal flap, with interrupted sutures for vertical incisions and interdental sutures between incisors.

A satisfactory long-term result can only be achieved when the dog's teeth are regularly brushed by the owner (Fig. 9–11).

Postoperative Care and Prophylaxis

After periodontal treatment, particularly after operations, administration of antibiotics is recommended for about a week. Teeth will clean themselves, provided the masticatory system functions adequately. Soft food rich in carbohydrates enhances plaque formation.

Mechanical Cleaning

The most effective prophylaxis is tooth brushing. Dog owners should be informed when their puppies are first vaccinated that dogs should become acquainted with tooth brushing. Puppies easily become accustomed to tooth brushing, but older dogs find it more difficult. A small child's toothbrush with rounded plastic bristles is recommended. One should use precipitated chalk, rather than a tooth paste with strong aromatic additions.

Chemotherapeutics

Chlorhexidine solutions are available. According to the patient's size and the degree of disease, a dose of ointment between the size of a pea and the size of a cherry is applied to the teeth and gingiva. The finger used to apply the ointment should be covered with a rubber finger protector because the water-insoluble ointment adheres to the skin. Once the ointment has been applied, its antibacterial effect will last longer than 12 hours because of the adherent properties of chlorhexidine. The ointment, which has a sticky consistency, protects the gingiva from irritants. After long-term application, chlorhexidine may cause brown stains, which can easily be removed by rubber polishers.

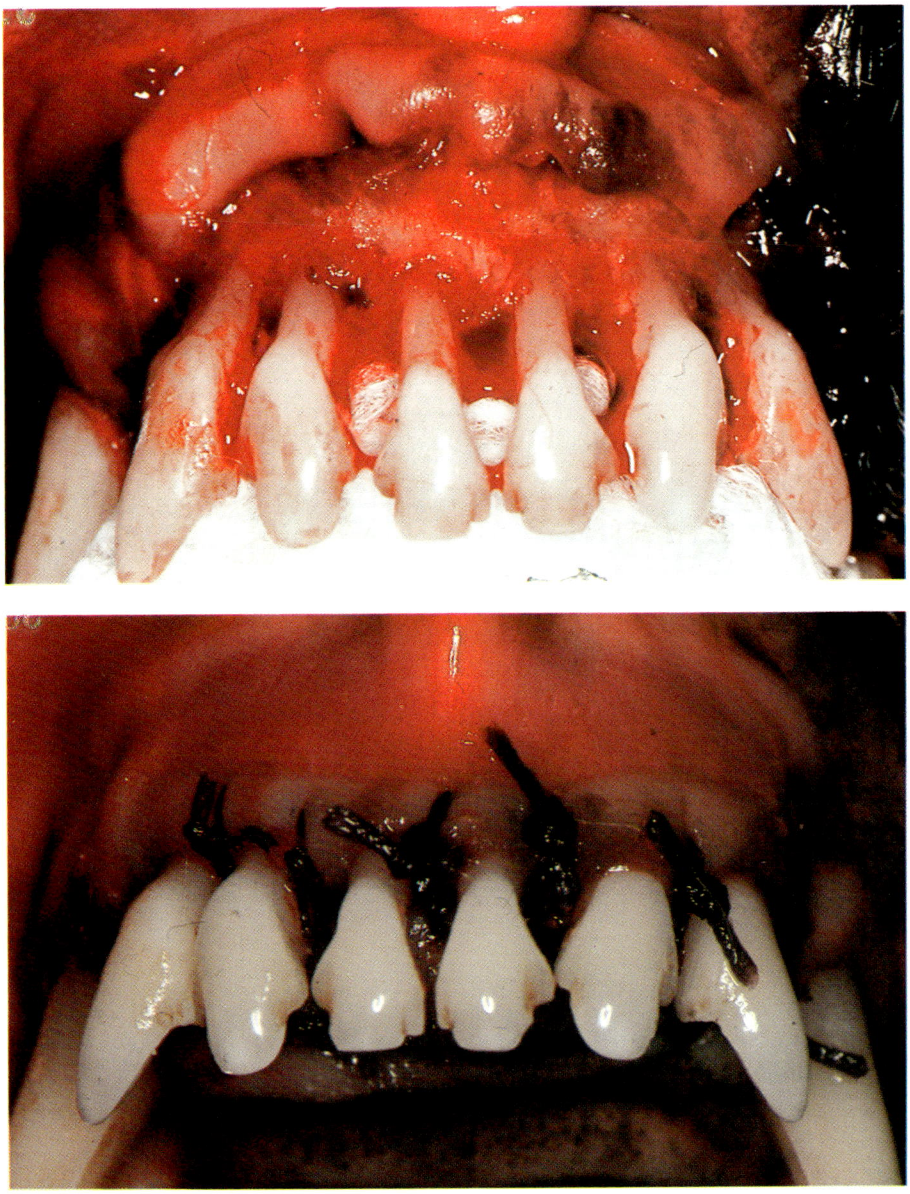

A

B

Fig. 9–11. Flap surgery in the maxillary incisor region in a 5-year-old poodle. *A,* Reflection of the mucoperiosteal flap. *B,* Repositioning and suturing after osteoplasty, cleaning, and polishing of tooth necks and roots.

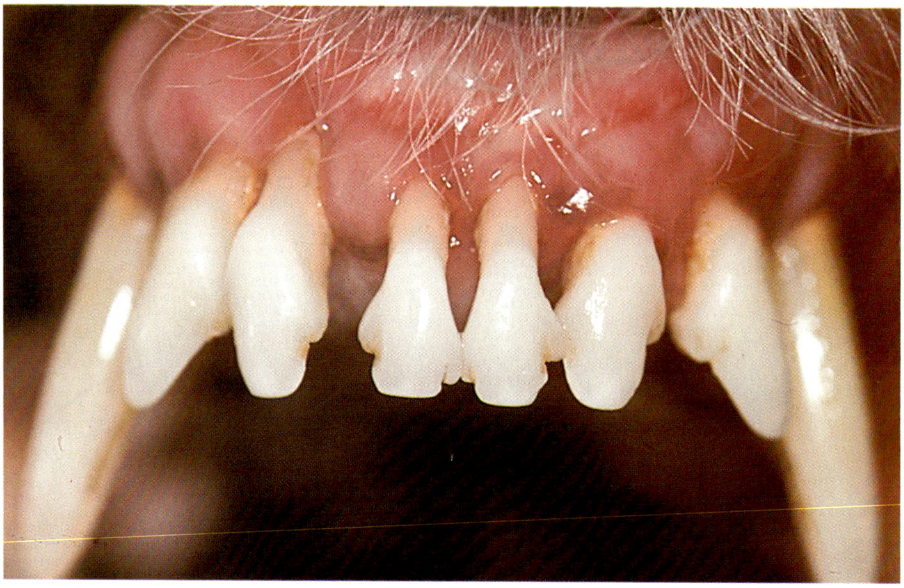

C

Fig. 9–11. ***Continued*** *C*, Follow-up a year later; regular tooth brushing by the owner has provided an excellent long-term result.

Feeding

Loosened teeth and a softened jaw bone are often caused by unnatural and wrong feeding. Excessive feeding of meat offal, known as the all-meat syndrome, leads to secondary alimentary hyperparathyroidism.

We recommend a daily oral dose of precipitated chalk of 1 teaspoon per 10 kg body weight per day. For prophylaxis, a change from conventional food to canned food has proved successful. Canned food has a balanced ratio of calcium to phosphorus, to prevent food-induced metabolic disturbances and to delay plaque formation.

PERIODONTOSIS (Primary Degenerative Periodontal Disease)

Signs and Symptoms

Periodontosis without concomitant inflammation is rare in dogs and does not occur in cats. A mixed form of periodontitis and periodontosis is common. Clinically, that these two diseases cannot be clearly distinguished is of secondary importance for treatment. The symptoms of periodontosis are loosening and migration of teeth (mesial movement).

Treatment

Because a combination of periodontitis and periodontosis is harmful, the formation of periodontitis should be prevented.

Prior to performing glass-fiber splinting, one should prepare the maxillary labial surfaces or the lingual surfaces of incisors by the acid-etch technique (see Chap. 7). A glass-fiber bundle is applied to the dried surfaces and is soaked with liquid composite (Fig. 9–12*A*). Glass fibers and resin have the same refractive index, and the hardened materials become transparent. To achieve sta-

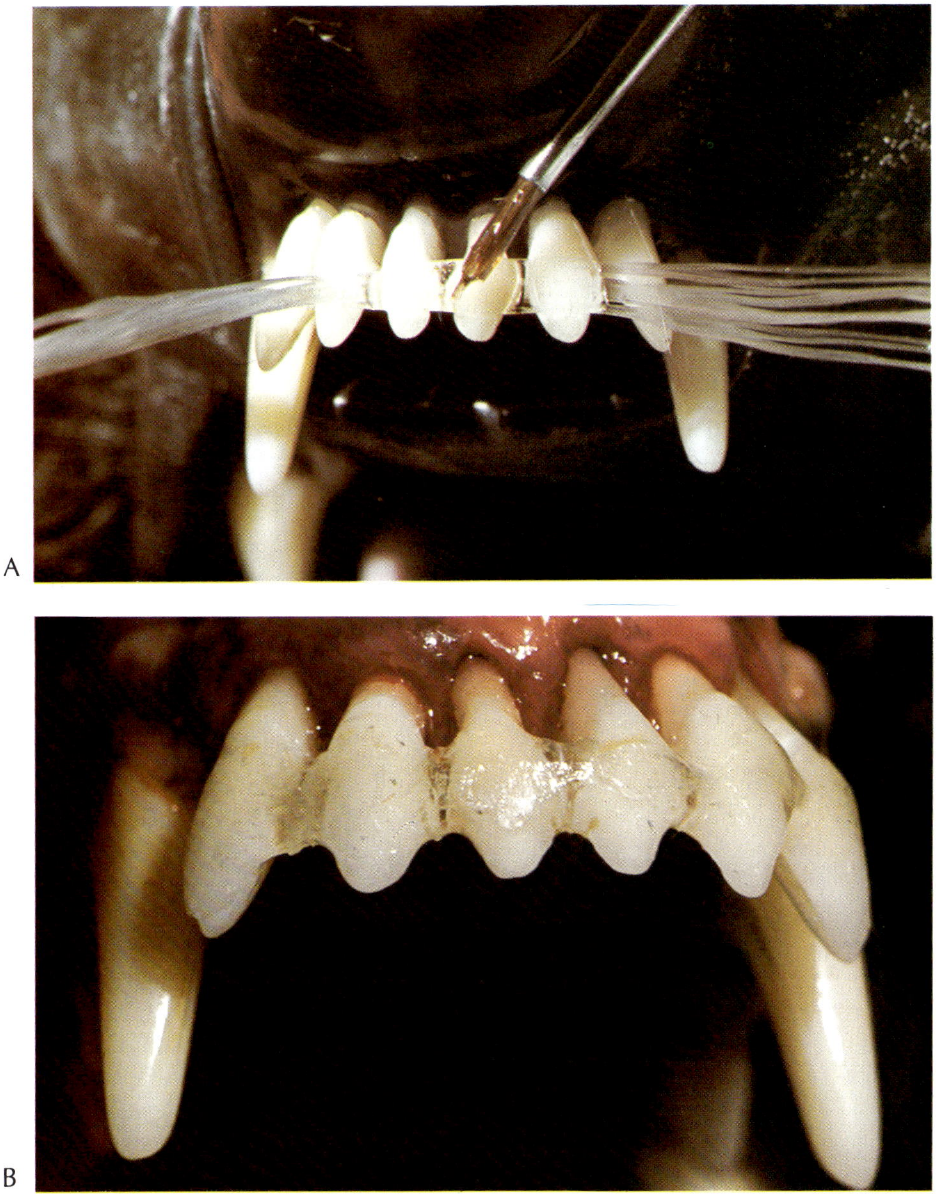

Fig. 9–12. Periodontosis. Stabilization of loosened teeth by means of a glass-fiber composite splint. *A,* Glass fibers are applied on the cleaned and etched incisors close to the contact points and are soaked with liquid composite. *B,* The glass-fiber and composite splint in the incisor region in a dog.

bility of the splint, several layers of liquid resin must be applied. The glass fibers that protrude over the ends of the bridge are cut off by rotary instruments or shears. These parts of the bridge must be coated with a thin layer of pasty composite, to protect the mucosa from possibly protruding glass-fiber points. Finally, a glossy sealant is applied (Fig. 9–12*B*).

By this time, the teeth have often stabilized themselves by temporary splint fixation. The splint can easily be removed with a high-speed handpiece and composite disks.

The patient's owner should be told to perform regular oral hygiene, in the form of tooth brushing, to prevent plaque and food debris from collecting in the interdental spaces.

HYPERPARATHYROIDISM

Pathogenesis

Tumors of the parathyroid glands are caused by an insufficiency of calcium or by an excess of phosphorus in the food (secondary alimentary hyperparathyroidism). Nephropathy (secondary renal hyperparathyroidism) or malfunction of the parathyroid gland may lead to a decalcification of the jaw (rubber jaw disease). This disease is frequently caused by unbalanced feeding (all-meat syndrome), which allow the surplus of phosphorus to stimulate the parathyroid gland. In parathyroid gland malfunction, calcium is removed first from the jaw and then progressively from the skull, the spine, the ribs, and finally, from the long bones.

Treatment

Mineral metabolism can be returned to normal by giving the patient lime, 1 teaspoon per 10 kg body weight per day. Food should have a well-balanced mineral content; canned food is recommended. The parenteral administration of calcium, vitamin AD_3E, and anabolic substances is another possibility.

IMMUNE-MEDIATED STOMATITIDES

The immune system of the oral cavity is complex. Although tremendous advances have been made in understanding these complexities, therapy remains only marginally effective. Success or failure in controlling the various stomatitides is in part related to the particular disease and its cause. The central issue in any therapeutic program is the control of plaque and calculus formation by both the veterinarian and the animal owner. At one end of the spectrum, in animals that are IgA deficient devastating periodontitis occurs, with massive alveolar bone necrosis (Fig. 9–13). These animals require complete tooth extraction; anything less compromises the integrity of the maxilla and the mandible. Postoperative antibiotic therapy aids in healing soft tissue. Animals that have recurring ulcerative stomatitis with moderate periodontitis respond to intensive dental prophylaxis and adjunct immunostimulation therapy.

The immunostimulation therapy includes Staphage lysate (phase-lysed staphylococci) and L-thyroxine. The dosage of Staphage lysate, injected at weekly intervals, is as follows: 0.1 ml interdermally; 0.2 ml subcutaneously; 0.3 ml subcutaneously; 0.4 ml subcutaneously; 0.5 ml subcutaneously; and then 0.5 ml weekly until the periodontitis is controlled. The time intervals between doses

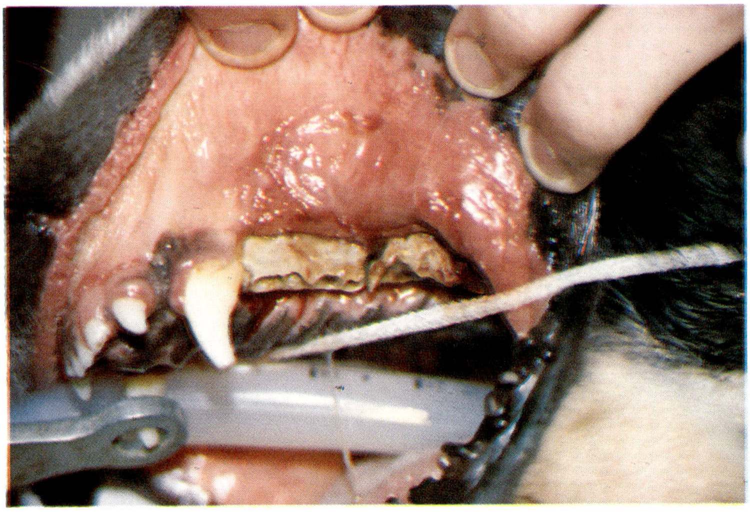

Fig. 9–13. IgA-deficient dog. Note the total necrosis of the gingiva with the resulting exposure and loss of maxillary alveolar bone.

is gradually increased in weekly increments for maintenance. In dogs that weigh more than 18 kg, the dose may be increased up to 1.5 ml Staphage lysate if the proper response has not been obtained. The dosage for L-thyroxine is 0.1 mg per 4.5 kg of body weight per day. The maximum dose is 0.5 mg per 4.5 kg body weight per day.

Animals with pemphigus lesions in the oral cavity respond to immunosuppressive doses of steroids or of special immunosuppressive agents, with the usual poor prognosis associated with this disease and therapy.

At the other end of the spectrum are the animals with varying degrees of allergic responses, such as atrophy, contact dermatitis, and inherent allergic dermatitis, that exacerbate a pre-existing periodontitis caused by owners' neglect. These animals respond better than others to therapy. Routine dental prophylaxis and education of the patient's owner restore the oral cavity to health.

SPECIAL DISEASES OF THE ORAL MUCOSA IN CATS

Plasmacytic Stomatitis

The presence of raspberry-like, red proliferations of the gingiva and oral mucosa is the diagnostic sign of this disorder. These lesions are liable to bleed, especially in the region of the mucolabial fold between the maxilla and the mandible (Fig. 9–14).

The cause is unknown. It may be a special granulomatous form of leukemia or an immunologic deficiency of lymphatic cells of the oral mucosa. Biopsy reveals heavy infiltration of plasmacytes.

Treatment

After treatment with antibiotics, the proliferations are dissected with a high-frequency electrosurgery unit; in less-advanced cases, a topical application of 50% trichloracetic acid solution is sufficient. The proliferations often recur within

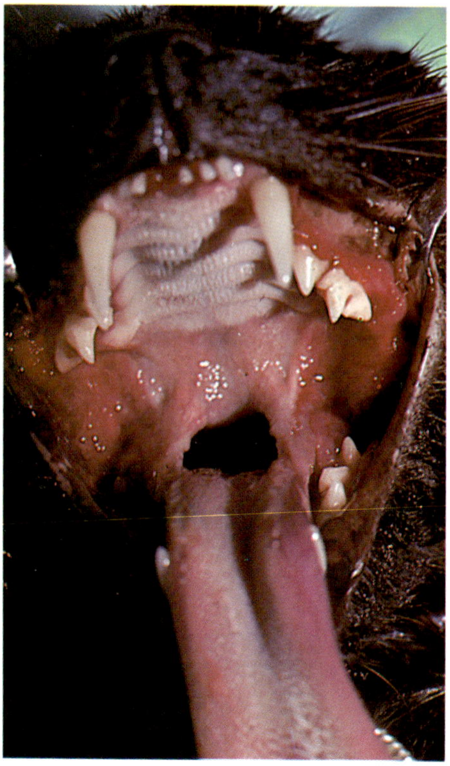

Fig. 9–14. Plasmacytic stomatitis complex in a cat. Note the raspberry-like proliferations at the gingival margin and at the mucolabial fold between the maxilla and the mandible.

a few weeks or months of initial treatment. Oral administration of steroids is then indicated for about 10 days. If the disease recurs, progestins should be administered orally. The next recurrence must be treated surgically. The prognosis is frequently poor.

Glossitis

The signs of glossitis are inflammation and thickening of the tongue, vesiculation on the sublingual mucosa, and ulceration in advanced cases. Glossitis is caused by viral infection and is treated with antibiotics, anabolic substances, and vitamins. Local treatment is the same as for gingivitis and periodontitis.

Stomatitis Plaut-Vincenti

This form of gingivitis and stomatitis is caused by fusobacteria and spirilla. It is considered a disease of animals in poor physical condition (insufficiency of defense mechanisms).

Treatment is with antibiotics, local topical applications, as in gingivitis and periodontitis, anabolic substances, and vitamins.

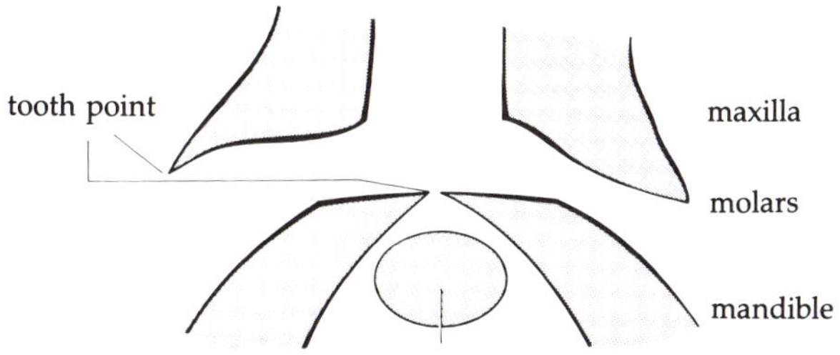

Fig. 9–15. Frequent dental anomalies in rodents include the formation of a sharp point and a bridge-like overgrowth in the mandible because of malpositioned teeth.

SPECIAL DISEASES IN RODENTS

Stomatitis is caused by the sharp points of malpositioned teeth. In the mandible, these points grow together and thus form a bridge above the tongue (Fig. 9–15). Malpositioned teeth have to be corrected repeatedly because the condition recurs.

Anorexia, exhaustion, loss of weight, and dry impacted food in the cheek pocket are the **symptoms and signs** of stomatitis in rodents.

The **treatment** of stomatitis consists of grinding the mandibular teeth with cylindric burs in a high-speed handpiece, cutting off the sharp points, and applying local astringents.

Loss of weight and anorexia may also occur in rodents with normal dentition. In such animals, the oral cavity is usually full of greenish, soft, thoroughly masticated food that cannot be swallowed; the cause of this condition is unknown.

DISEASES OF THE ORAL CAVITY IN REPTILES

Necrotizing ulcerative gingivitis, or fusopirillosis, in snakes is caused by fusobacteria and spirilla. The **symptoms and signs** are anorexia, mouth odor, and

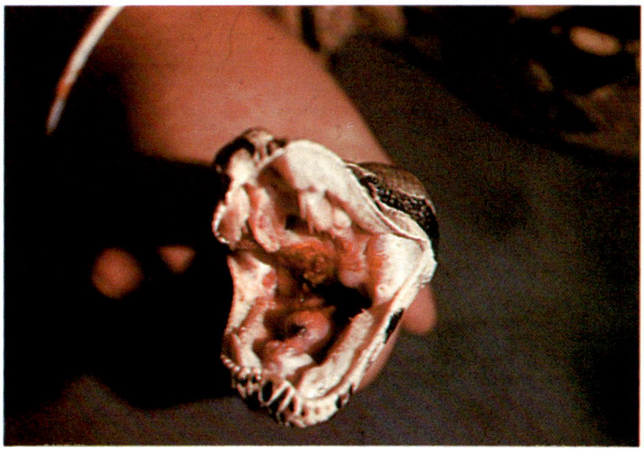

Fig. 9–16. Necrotizing ulcerative gingivitis (fusospirillosis) in a snake.

yellowish membranous coatings (Fig. 9–16). **Treatment** consists of topical application of chlorhexidine, trypaflavine (acriflavine hydrochloride), and trichloracetic acid.

Poisonous snakes should be put in a refrigerator for 20 to 30 minutes. Because of the cold, they are nearly immobile and can be managed easily.

Bibliography: 3, 6, 11, 24, 34, 40, 43, 49, 51, 56, 58, 60, 62, 64

10

Physiologic and Irregular Wear

PHYSIOLOGIC WEAR

The cuspal enamel teeth in carnivores, as well as the incisors in herbivores, finish growing shortly after eruption. Tooth substance lost by physiologic or irregular wear is not replaced.

The extent of physiologic wear depends on the hard tooth tissue and on the consistency of the animal's food. Altogether, the physiologic abrasion in carnivores is insignificant; it is most noticeable at the incisors and the anterior premolars. These teeth have an outer white enamel ring, an intermediate ring of dentin, and, in the center, the pulp cavity, which is visible as a dark spot. The slight tooth abrasion occurring in pigs can be ignored because of their short life expectancy.

Abrasion of the incisors in horses is 2 mm per year, and that of the posterior teeth is about 3 to 4 mm per year. Physical constitution and breed play an important part; for example, Lipizzaners have a much stronger and harder dentin than any other breed.

More abrasion is caused by feeding hard, dry food mixed with dirt, sand, or grain husks. The central enamel niches of the incisors and maxillary posterior teeth disappear first; the outer enamel ring is preserved longest. The central dentin is abraded flatly. Senile excavation begins to develop during the eighteenth year of life.

The softer dentin and cementum are abraded more quickly than the hard enamel. This process leaves an oval enamel ring with a serrated elevation in the posterior teeth or an oval-to-round enamel ring in the incisors. Thus, the teeth of herbivores maintain the surface structure necessary for chewing hard food.

The enamel-folded teeth in herbivores grow for a longer period of time and compensate abrasion until tooth growth stops; the posterior teeth of horses continue growing up to the sixth or seventh year of life. Later, up to the fifteenth year of life, the tooth is pushed out by bone apposition at the bottom of the alveolus. Finally, the rest of the tooth bulk is used for mastication by resorbing the bony alveolar margin. At that time, hyperplasia of the root cementum causes a slight elongation.

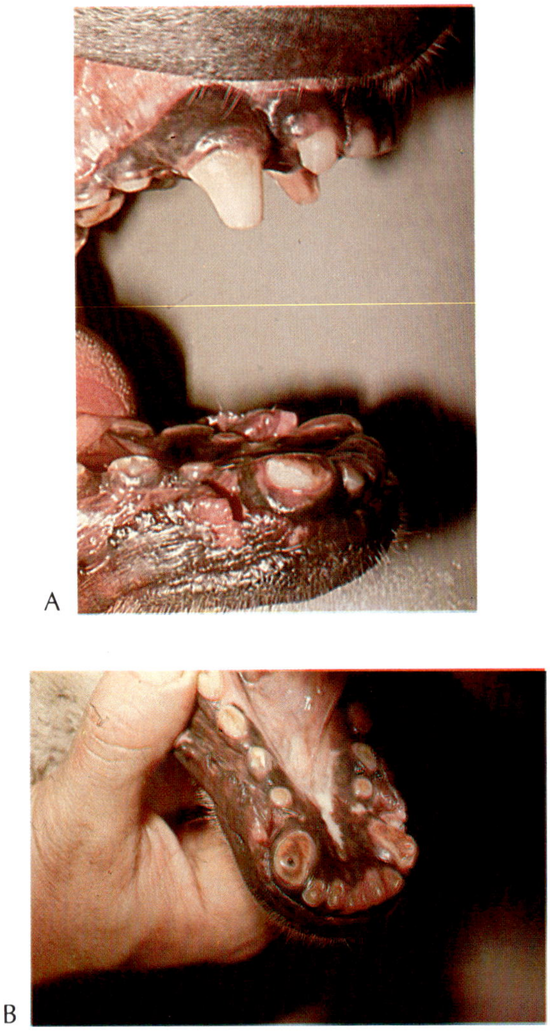

Fig. 10–1. *A* and *B,* Excessive abrasion of dentition in a dog ("stone biter").

Excavation of posterior teeth in cows starts between the ages of 14 and 16 years. A 25- to 30-year-old horse has only superficially anchored teeth resting in its jaw. Within the dentin layer, brown spots become more visible as abrasion progresses; these brown spots are formed by the receding pulp.

Horses chew in such a way that the mandible is moved laterally and then back to its central position under pressure. These repeated lateral movements are greatest when the horse is eating hay, less when the horse is eating oats, and least when the horse is eating bran or mashed oats. Mastication starts in the premolar region and continues in the molar region. When the food has been thoroughly mixed with saliva, it is swallowed.

Ruminants chew their food when it has been softened in the rumen, thus lessening mastication pressure at the posterior teeth.

IRREGULAR WEAR

Dogs that are fed bones regularly, undergo extensive attack training, or play with stones or other hard objects show greater wear of the incisors, canines, and premolars than other dogs (Fig. 10–1). All these teeth are finally abraded to round or oval tooth remnants with dark spots of secondary dentin in their centers. These tooth remnants are firmly anchored in the sound jaws. Excessively abraded teeth need not be treated; owners should try to change their dogs' habits, as well as the kind of food their dogs eat.

Irregular wear can be noted on the distal surfaces of the canines and incisors in dogs that bite the metal bars of their cages or garden fences (Fig. 10–2*A*). Such dogs are called "cage biters." The occurrence of such defects is mainly restricted to the following: (1) military and police dogs; (2) dogs belonging to professional breeders; and (3) dogs kept in gardens surrounded by iron fences. These changes should not be mistaken for enamel hypoplasia.

Local defects may cause tooth fractures and should be either filled with TMS-pin-anchored amalgam (Fig. 10–2*B* and *C*) or coated with a composite or steel crown. Irregular wear is rare in cats.

In the United States, especially in Nebraska, irregular tooth wear has occurred in cattle because of the short, hard grass that is mixed with sand. Treatment consists of tooth capping with steel crowns.

Sharp Points

When horses eat mechanically prepared food, in the form of pellets of mashed food, over a long period, the chewing motions diminish in their lateral extent. Because of this change, the teeth in the narrower mandible are abraded primarily on their buccal surfaces, and the teeth in the maxilla are abraded primarily on their lingual surfaces. Consequently, sharp points are formed on the buccal surfaces of the maxillary teeth and on the lingual surfaces of the mandibular teeth. These points lead to painful lesions of the buccal mucosa or the tongue and cause a masticatory disorder.

The symptoms of this disorder are excessive salivation, prolonged food intake, foul mouth odor, and so-called "quidding." Coarse food is constantly moved in the cheek pocket until cigar-shaped food bars about 10 cm in length are formed. The horse drops these "quids," which are then found in or beside the crib. Unchewed oat grains can be found in the feces. Unilateral or bilateral

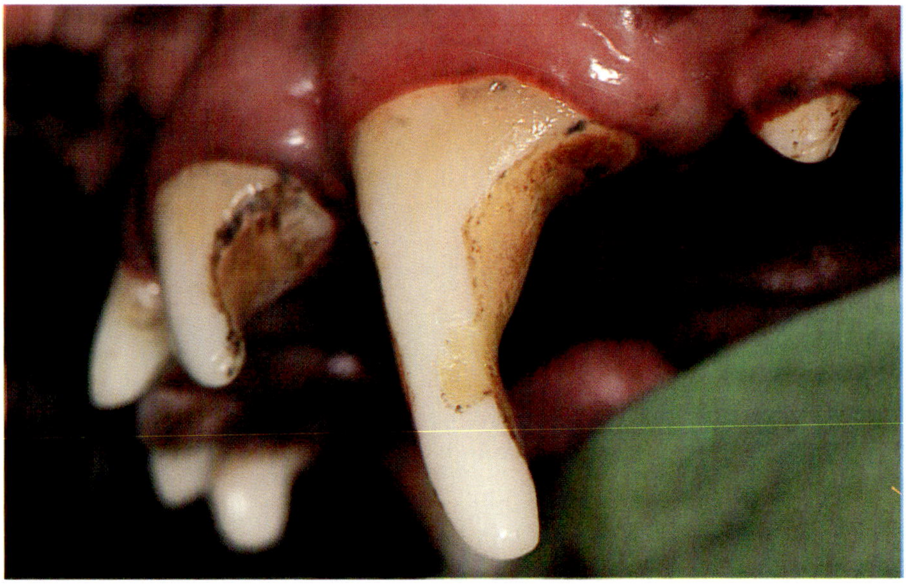

A

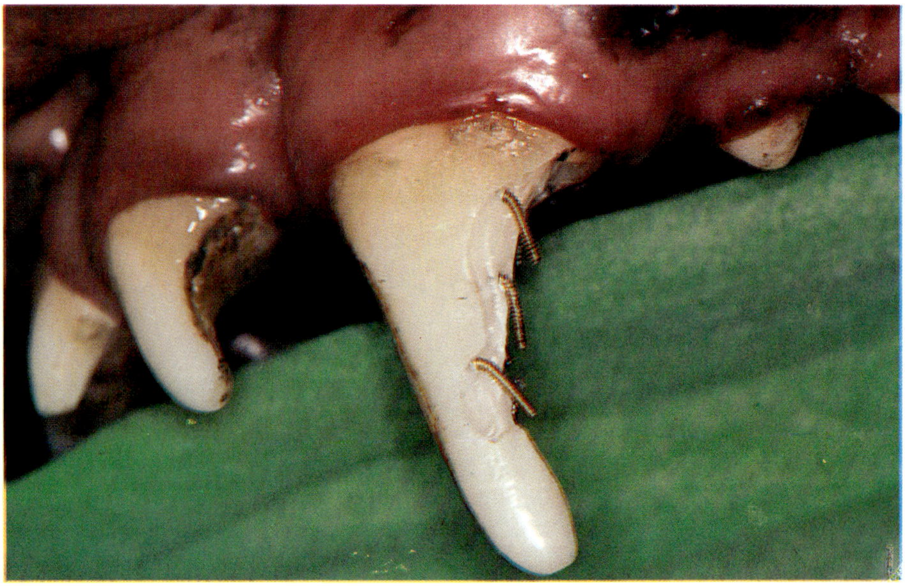

B

Fig. 10–2. *A,* Irregular wear, localized at the distal surfaces of a canine tooth and an incisor (I3). *B,* Flat dovetail preparation and inserted Thread-Mate-System pins.

C 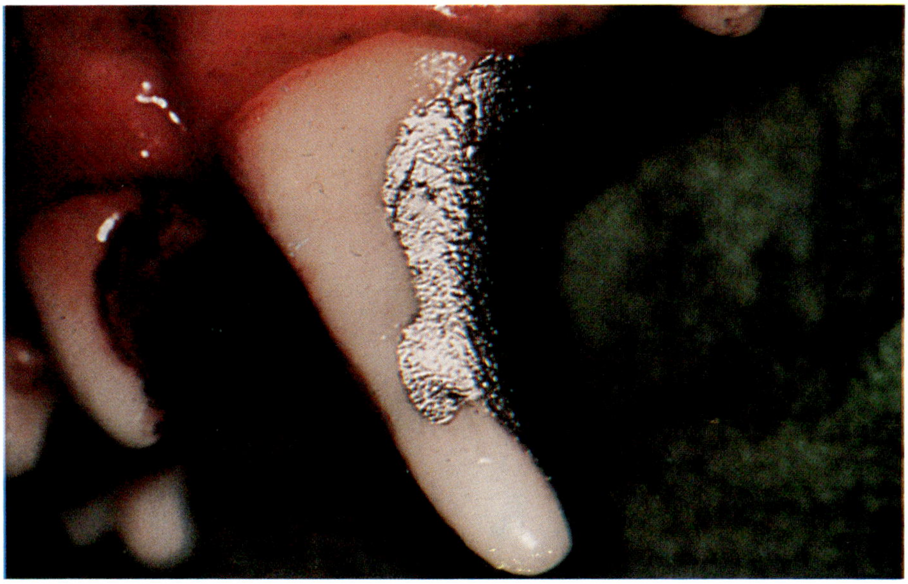

Fig. 10–2. *Continued* *C*, Filling with silver amalgam.

atrophy of the masticatory muscles may also occur. Cachexia, diarrhea, and colic are occasional symptoms.

Treatment

The sharp points are ground off with a hand rasp or an electric grinder. Excessive grinding should be avoided, to preserve a normal occlusal surface. This treatment should be repeated at regular intervals. The animal should be fed coarser, less mashed food. Treatment can be performed on a standing horse; quiet horses need not be sedated. The best position for treatment is when the animal is standing with its hindquarters in a corner, with its head held by two assistants at the ears and halter. At the same time, one of the assistants holds the mouth wedge, which is inserted between the posterior teeth and cannot be thrown out as easily as a mouth lattice. If any sedation is necessary, xylazine should not be used because of the head-drop effect.

When handpieces are used, the horse must be in lateral recumbency for safety; the animal's neck should be positioned higher than the mouth, to guarantee the runoff of cooling water, saliva, and blood. A treatment box could be used for the sedated but standing horse.

Shear Mouth

Shear mouth is a long-lasting, unilateral masticatory disturbance that causes painful inflammation of a jaw joint, unilateral jaw fracture, unilateral toothache, or painful mucosal irritation and allows only the occlusal surfaces of the posterior teeth in the faultless part of the jaw to make full contact. The posterior teeth in the faulty part of the jaw are worn off on the inner top and the outer lower surfaces; two sharp-edged rows of teeth thereby develop. These teeth glide past each other, and the points lacerate the gingiva and the palate, respectively.

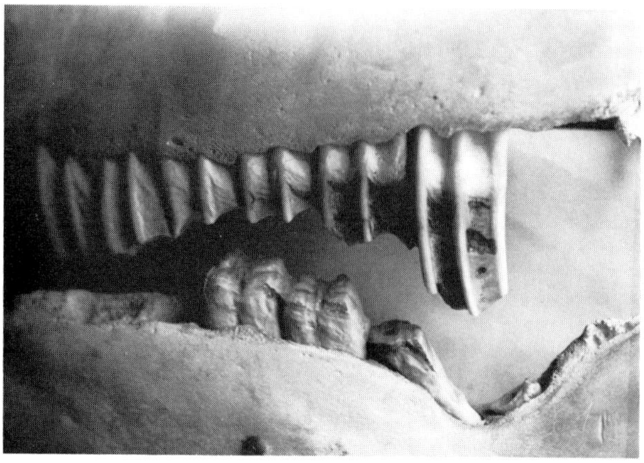

Fig. 10–3. Uneven occlusal surfaces caused by a loss of mandibular posterior teeth.

Consequently, painful stomatitis, osteomyelitis, or loosening of teeth may occur. Unilateral atrophy of masticatory muscles is common.

In many cases, even the incisors are abraded at an oblique angle. The general symptoms correspond to those described in the discussion of sharp points in horses' teeth.

Treatment

As far as possible, the faults should be eliminated. When treated locally, the horse should be in lateral recumbency. The projecting teeth and tooth points are trimmed with sharp shears or a handpiece; the occlusion of posterior teeth treated in this way should then be normal. Treatment should be repeated when necessary.

Wave Mouth and Step Mouth

The loss of a posterior tooth, greater abrasion of one or more teeth because of hypoplasia or fracture, or an uneven occlusal surface causes a weaker abrasion of the antagonist or antagonists, which project farther than the adjacent teeth

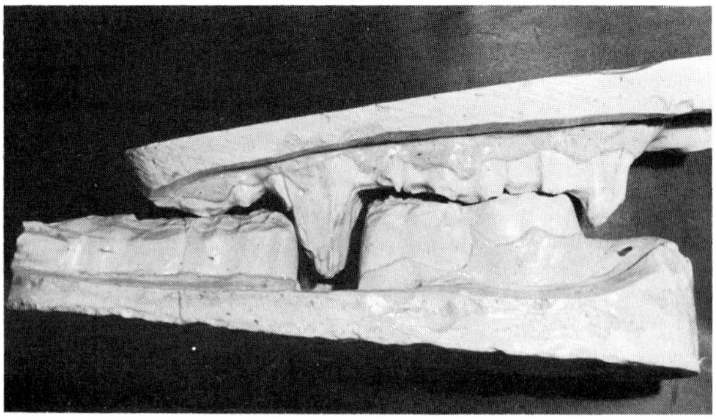

Fig. 10–4. Cast of exsuperantia dentis in a horse. A chisel-shaped tooth (P2) is growing into an interdental space (diastema). Note the incongruity of the occlusal surfaces.

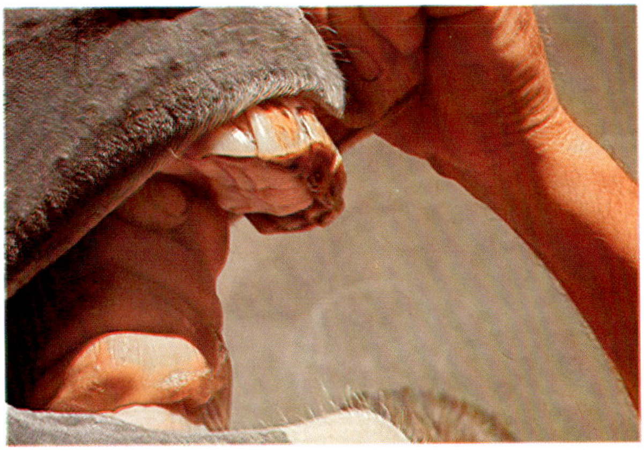

Fig. 10–5. Obliquely abraded incisors in a cribbing horse.

(Fig. 10–3). If a tooth grows into an interdental space, it takes the shape of a chisel and projects farther than the other teeth (Fig. 10–4).

A group of projecting teeth is trimmed to a rounded prominence that forms a congruent indentation in the opposing row of teeth. Elongated teeth or groups of teeth cause painful indentations or purulent osteomyelitis in the soft tissue and bone of the opposing jaw and may result in severe disturbance of mastication and food intake.

Treatment consists of cutting off projecting teeth with shears or trimming them at annual intervals. In the premolar region, bridging the diastema or filling a cemental hypoplasia with inlay could be considered.

Abnormal Wear Due to Cribbing

Cribbing horses bite the edge of the crib or other projections; another common bad habit in horses is the constant rubbing of the incisors along the crib.

The sign of a cribbing disorder is the wearing of the anterior surfaces of the incisors at an oblique angle, to reveal the pulp cavity (star), which is ordinarily sealed by secondary dentin. This disorder primarily occurs in the maxillary incisors in cribbing horses and may complicate the estimation of the animal's age (Fig. 10–5).

Bibliography: 4, 5, 11, 18, 47

Bibliography

1. Adams D, Gillespie J. Restoration of an incisor tooth of a wolfhound: case report. J. Small Anim Pract 1979; 20:691.
2. Autalovska Z. Zahnschäden durch Tetrazykline. Pro Medico 1977; 46:18.
3. Bartels P. Zahnbehandlung beim Hund. Tierärztl Prax 1973; 1:437.
4. Becker E. Neuzeitliche Zahnbehandlung beim Pferd. Hannover: H Schaper, 1938.
5. Becker E. In: Joest E. Handbuch der speziellen pathologischen Anatomie der Haustiere, 3rd ed (vol 5). Berlin: Paul Parey, 1970.
6. Bell AF. Dental disease in the dog. J Small Anim Pract 1966; 6:421.
7. Bellizzi R, Worsin J, Woody RD, Keller DL., Drorotij E. Nonsurgical endodontic therapy, utilizing lingual coronal access on the mandibular canine tooth of dogs. J Am Vet Med Assoc 1981; 179:370.
8. Berge E, Westhues M. Tierärztliche Operationslehre, 29th ed. Berlin: Paul Parey, 1969.
9. Bigler B. Experimentelle und klinische Untersuchungen zur Frage der endodontischen Therapie des Hundegebisses. Zentralbl Veterinarmed (A) 1978; 25:794.
10. Bodingbauer J. Zahnfrakturen beim Hund. Wien Tierärztl Wochenschr 1947; 34:447.
11. Bodingbauer J. In: Wirth D. Lexikon der praktischen Therapie und Prophylaxe für Tierärzte (vol 2). Vienna: Urban and Schwarzenberg, 1956.
12. Bodingbauer J, Hager G. Zur Frage der Ätiologie der Zahnunterzahl (Oligodontie) des Hundes. Wien Tierärztl Wochenschr 1959; 46:213, 313.
13. Bodingbauer J. Hochgradige Zahnunterzahl (Aplasie) beim Hund. Wien Tierärztl Wochenschr 1974; 61:301.
14. van den Brink FH. Die Säugetiere Europas, 2nd ed. Hamburg: Paul Parey, 1968.
15. Charnock M, Usher JJ. Fitting a prosthetic crown to a canine tooth in a police dog. Vet Rec 1968; 83:464.
16. Claus C, Grobben K. Lehrbuch der Zoologie, 9th ed. Marburg: Elwertsche Verlagsbuchhandlung, 1917.
17. Colmery B. In: Bojrab MJ. Pathophysiology in Small Animal Surgery (vol 2). Philadelphia: Lea & Febiger, 1983.
18. Dietz O, Schaetz F, Schleiter M, Teuscher R. Anästhesie und Operationen bei Grossund Kleintieren, 2nd ed. Stuttgart: Enke, 1978.
19. Dobberstein J, Koch T. Lehrbuch der vergleichenden Anatomie der Haustiere (vol 2). Leipzig: Hirzel, 1954.
20. Eisenmenger E. Die Zahnfachentzündung des Jungpferdes, ihre Ursachen und operative Behandlung unter Ehrhaltung des vollständigen Gebisses. Wien Tierärztl Wochenschr 1959; 46:51.
21. Eisenmenger E. Konservative Behandlung von Zahnfrakturen des Hundes. Wien Tierärztl Wochenschr 1971; 58:30.
22. Ellenberger-Baum. Handbuch der vergleichenden Anatomie der Haustiere, 18th ed. Berlin: Springer, 1943.
23. Firth LK. In: Kirk. Current Veterinary Therapy, 5th ed. Philadelphia, WB Saunders, 1974.
24. Fritsch R, Salek M. Über die Parodontitis des Hundes. Berl Münch Tierärztl Wochenschr 1966; 77:478.
25. Gardner A, Darke PH, Keary GT. Dental caries in domesticated dogs. J Am Vet Med Assoc 1962; 140:433.
26. Gass H. Affen in der Kleintierpraxis. Kleintierpraxis 1978; 23:127.
27. Grzimek B. Grzimeks Tierleben, Enzyklopädie des Tierreichs (11 vols). Zurich: Kindler, 1969.
28. Grzimek B. Grzimeks Tierleben, Enzyklopädie des Tierreichs (12 vols). Zurich: Kindler, 1972.
29. Hamilton CJ, Ridgway RL. Dowel and core preparation and full gold coverage of maxillary canine teeth in a German shepherd. VM/SAC 1976; 71:176.
30. Jaksch W, Glawischnig E. Klinische Propädeutik der inneren Krankheiten der Haustiere (Parey Student Text No 5). Berlin: Paul Parey, 1976.
31. Jirava E, et al.: Über die Behandlung von frakturierten Zahnen bei Hunden Berl Münch Tierärztl Wochenschr 1966; 79:235.

32. Joest E. Handbuch der speziellen pathologischen Anatomie der Haustiere, 3rd ed (vol 5). Berlin: Paul Parey, 1967.
33. Krölling O, Grau H. Lehrbuch der Histologie und vergleichenden mikroskopischen Anatomie der Haustiere. Berlin: Paul Parey, 1960.
34. Kühn A. Grundriss der allgemeinen Zoologie, 15th ed. Stuttgart: Thieme, 1964.
35. Meyer R, Suter G. Epidemiologische Untersuchungen am Hundegebiss. Schweiz Arch Tierheilkd 1976; 118:308.
36. Mooser M. Zahnärztlich vergleichende Untersuchungen an 425 Hundeschädeln. Schweiz Arch Tierheilkd 1958; 100:209.
37. Nickel R, Schummer A, Seiferle E. Lehrbuch der Anatomie der Haustiere (vol 2: Eingeweide). Berlin: Paul Parey, 1960.
38. Ramy CT, Segreto VA. Apicoectomy and root canal therapy for exposed pulp canal in the dog. J Am Vet Med Assoc 1967; 150:977.
39. Ridgway RL, Zielke DR. Nonsurgical endodontic technique for dogs. J Am Vet Med Assoc 1979; 174:82.
40. Ross DL, Meyers JW. Endodontic therapy for canine teeth in the dog. J Am Vet Med Assoc 1970; 157:1713.
41. Ross DL. In: Bojrab MJ. Current Techniques in Small Animal Surgery (vol 1). Philadelphia: Lea & Febiger, 1975.
42. Rubin LD, Maplesden DC, Singer RR. Root canal therapy in dogs. VM/SAC 1978; 73:593.
43. Schlup D. Epidemiologische und morphologische Untersuchungen am Katzengebiss. Dissertation, University of Bern, 1981.
44. Schmeltzer LD, Carolan RJ, Ohta RM. Use of conventional endodontic therapy in a case of veterinary medicine. J Am Dent Assoc 1980; 100:218.
45. Schneck GW. Caries in the dog. J Am Vet Med Assoc 1976; 150:1142.
46. Schulze W, Konrad H. Zur konservierenden Zahnheilkunde in der Hundepraxis. Berl Münch Tierärztl Wochenschr 1955; 68:338, 353, 369.
47. Selhorst F. Orthodontische und kieferorthopädische Behandlungen und Versuche an Hunden. Dissertation, University of Munich, 1964.
48. Sevcik F. X-ray examination of changes in the alveolus produced by extraction of an intact tooth in the dog. Veterinarstvi 1971; 21:465.
49. Silbersiepe-Berge U. Müller. Lehrbuch der speziellen Chirurgie fur Tierärzte und Studierende, 15th ed. Stuttgart: Enke, 1976.
50. Spannbrucker D, Schmidtke D, Schmidtke HO. Anomalien der Backenzähne bei Zwerkaninchen und Meerschweinchen. Kleintierpraxis 1977; 22:331.
51. Studer E, Stapley RB. The role of dry foods in maintaining healthy teeth and gums in the cat. VM/SAC 1973; 68:1124.
52. Stülpnagel M, Becker B. Zur Technik des Beschleifens von Backenzähnen bei Nagern. Kleintierpraxis 1978; 23:395.
53. Sweetman AJ. Traumatic incisor injuries in small animals. J Small Anim Pract 1973; 14:715.
54. Taylor RA III, Raymond P. Endodontia in the dog. VM/SAC 1972; 67:1197.
55. Tholen MA. The veterinary dental record: key to veterinary dental medicine. VM/SAC 1983; 78:1403.
56. Tober-Mayer B. Vorschläge zur Narkose bei Kaninchen, Meerschweinchen und kleinen Nagern. Kleintierpraxis 1977; 22:335.
57. Triaden H. Tierzahnheilkunde: Zahnerhaltung (Füllungs therapie mit "Composite Materials" und Endodontie) bei Affen und Raubtieren. Schweiz Arch Tierheilkd 1972; 114:292.
58. Triadan H. Parodontologie bei Affen und Raubtieren. Schweiz Arch Tierheilkd 1973; 115:401.
59. Triska W. Experimentelle Studien über die Beisskraft. Pflügers Arch 1924; 204:660.
60. Wright JG. Some observations on dental disease in the dog. Vet Rec 1939; 51:408.
61. Wynn WP, Tremain LM, Mathews JR Jr. Restoration of a fractured canine tooth in a dog. J Am Vet Med Assoc 1973; 162:396.
62. Zetner K. Die prothetische Versorgung von Zahnfrakturen mit Adhäsivkunststoff. Kleintierpraxis 1976; 21:271.
63. Zetner K. Parodontopathien beim Kleintier. Kleintierpraxis 1977; 22:311.
64. Zetner K. Veterinary Stomatology. Folia Latina Veterinaria, 1979.
65. Zietzschmann O, Krölling O. Lehrbuch der Entwicklungsgeschichte der Haustiere. Berlin: Paul Parey, 1955.

Index

Page numbers followed by *f* indicate figures, numbers followed by *t* indicate tables.